Who's Afraid of Parkinson's?

The Finnish Association of Non-fiction Writers has supported the writing of this book.

Timo Montonen

Who's Afraid of Parkinson's?

My First Ten Hilarious Years

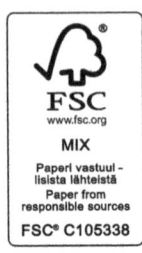

Publisher: BoD™ – Books on Demand, Helsinki, Finland

Manufacturer:
Books on Demand GmbH, Norderstedt. Germany

ISBN 978-952-330-095-8

Table of Content

"I'll tell you in this book, how I climbed a ladder, rose higher and higher step by step, toward the all sanctifying Parkinson's crown."

- Foreword

- Organizations, Projects, Websites

- Is There an Editor in this Book?

"**Oiva** *A club for early onset and people with Parkinson's at working age. I was crucial important to the birth and rouse of Oiva, and vice versa, from 2010 to 2014.*"

1. Foreword

I am translating from Finnish to English and at the same time editing the English version of this book. I have a pile of texts, which I have published in newspapers, social media and books from the year 2006 to 2015. The titles of my earlier books containing Parkinson's stories would be in English *Author's Book* (2008/2010/2015), *Towards a Better Life* (2011) and *I have Parkinson's, and I'm Proud of* it (2014). Sounds very positive or what you think? The last title, of course, is ironic, as you immediately realized.

About my English I would make a notification. Despite the fact, that I have learned English at various schools and at the university fifteen years all together and watched English movies over fifty years, I have used both Google and Microsoft Translators when needed. I do not hesitate to make lingual mistakes. Errors confirm that this is my personal story. There is a saying, that an error is the beginning of wisdom (or similar idiom in English?). Once when I was tutoring the top leaders of a big energy company, I tried to convince them that an error is a message. It is a message that should be heard and interpreted and from that base turn to learning and developing. But I don't aim to errors, I don't have to. They come without efforts, but the main point here is to become understood. This is what a Malaysian **Samuel Ng**, whom I had met in Montreal, Canada, at the 3rd World Parkinson Congress October 2013, wrote me in Facebook, when he suggested that I should write to him an English version of my first book about Parkinson's. So, thanks him that this book exists.

I do not always tell the writing or publishing date of a certain publication, because I've edited, as I said, the writings for this book and written a lot of new things, varying from minor details to wider summaries. Old posts, read and forgotten, have been the springboard for fresh ideas, the restoration of forgotten memories, loose details compassing to the integration so that the crumbs are structured an entity.

I'll tell you in this book, how I climbed a ladder, rose higher and higher step by step, toward the all sanctifying Parkinson's crown. I flew toward an illusion, preceded in carrying out voluntary work and of the disease as like marking the boxes in a school experiment, conquered kilometer square of invalidity and influencing one after the other.

I remember how soon after getting the diagnosis I joined the Parkinson's Association of Southern Finland (PASF). I remember how I inquired the similarities and differences of numerous local clubs which were part of nearly twenty areal associations which made up the national Finnish Parkinson's Association. I remember how I tried to understand the meaning of quite massive hierarchical organization, when there were only seven or eight thousand members in the areal associations. I remember how I travelled through a simulation of nearby future; how I saw in my mind a cavalcade of positions of trust and of responsibility in various levels. I decided that one day I would be the chairman of a local club, a member of the board of directors in the areal association and in the national association, and, of course, a union representative.

The fact that my Parkinson activity would take me from Helsinki, Finland, to London, UK, and to Montreal, Canada, in order to attend international meetings, never came in my mind. Neither did the fact that I would become gainfully employed in the association of my own disease. But so it was, when I dared to trust my ideas and apply for funding for new innovative activities – and give my own money, when the pleasure and benefit were near enough each other, such as the Canadian journey, so that before the 3rd World Parkinson's Congress I went with my daughter to Niagara Falls and pop star **Justin Bieber's** hometown Stratford...

But be patience, I'll tell all in time.

"Soon I noticed, that the Editor created a feeling of fiction."

2. Organizations, Projects, Websites

Here is a list of organizations I've been working with, projects I've been involved with, websites I've been writing to and some other concepts important in my Parkinson scene:

- **1HOURMORE** A project of EPDA together with Italian Publisher, writer and medical company. 2015. Lizi Graham, Director of Fundraising and Global Communications, asked me to attend.

- **444 Parkinson's Traveler** A project of Marcus Cranston. I answered to Marcus in Facebook and took responsibility in Finland. Spring 2014.

- **APC** Advocates for Parkinson Committee. I offered to become an Ambassador of WPC2016, next day I was asked to join the APC. Spring 2014-to Autumn 2016.

- **dg** Diagnosis

- **EPDA** European Parkinson's Disease Association. Important international context to me especially 2011-2013, but later too.

- **FPA** Finnish Parkinson's Association. I've done co-operation since 2007.

- **Oiva** A club for early onset and people with Parkinson's at working age. I was crucial important to the birth and rouse of Oiva, and vice versa, from 2010 to 2014.

- **Palmenia Writing Program** My job for fifteen years at the University of Helsinki , 2000-2015.

- **Parkinson's at Work site** A web site created in the PW from the base of my ideas. 2012.

- **Parkinson Place/Stop** A social media, where I met angry opponents 2010-2014.

- **PASF** Parkinson's Association of Southern Finland, the areal association I belong to, joined 2005.

- **Parkinson's at Work project** Two years project I planned and made true with Anna-Maria Salonen, a part-time project worker, 2012-2013

- **PD** Parkinson's disease

- **pwp** person with Parkinson's, people with Parkinson's.

- **Seminar on Parkinson's Disease and Working Life** An important public whole day event of the PW. Spring 2013.

- **Summer Wind** The Special Training Center of Finnish Parkinson's Association.

- **WPC** Word Parkinson Coalition/Congress.

- **WPC2013** 3rd World Parkinson Congress, Montreal, Canada, 2013.

- **WPC2016** 4th World Parkinson Congress, Portland, Oregon, USA2016.

3. Is There an Editor in this Book?

At some point of writing this book I began to imagine an Editor, who would comment my text. Maybe the writing process was too long and lonely. I had no-one to talk about it thoroughly. And yes, maybe I was a bit scared what would be the result, because I worked with foreign language without traditional publisher's aid in editing and marketing.

Soon I noticed, that the Editor created a feeling of fiction. The whole package began to be like a novel, and that was not what I intended to do. For all that, I was hesitating, I took the Editor's remarks away, and next day put them back.

Now I've come to a conclusion, that I give you, reader, as a literal gift some of the remarks of unknown Editor. I hope you have a couple of minutes time to this side path.

- You are reading the fragments I was able to collect from various sources after Timo, our brother in Parkinson's, deleted all his manuscripts, notes and computers and then simply vanished in the meaningless desert of an unbearable boredom, of which we healthy people don't want to know. His snoring is no longer with us, neither his obsessions, poor jokes nor forgetting other people's affairs immediately after hearing them. - *Editor*

- As far as I know the fragments are authentic, in the sense we can consider in this situation, where everything Timo left behind is from a second or third (or fourth and so on) source. - *Editor*

- While wanting to offer the readers as readable and coherent book as possible (books are expensive and you got to get a valuable piece of art for your money) I have edited the texts with tender touch. That's what Timo would have been wanted if he had thought this matter thoroughly. So, when you find Timo commenting this book in following chapters, you can be pretty sure that the comments origins to my editorial work. There was, I am sure, no this kind of book that Timo intended to create, if he was creating a book at all. - *Editor*

- Timo newer wanted this book in day light. But I see no choice than take the responsibility to collect, edit, write and publish this essential masterpiece of autobiographical contemplations. So, I publish this book against the will of Timo. So did **Max Brod**, who saved and edited the works of **Franz Kafka** after his death and let them become an infinite part of the granite base of Western Literature. Comparing Kafka to Timo is an act of honoring, and I'm honestly assured, that Kafka would have appreciated it. – *Editor*

- Humor? Irony? [Two vague words, unreadable.]

- Why did Timo write this kind of text? Or… Did he really write it? Was he in balance in his mind? Obviously not. If you compare this to other texts surrounding it, it's a kind of anomaly, like a punch to nose of everyone Timo is working with. Did he imagine, that he could continue co-operation usually, as nothing had happened? I guess he did! – *Editor*

- If Timo would have written and published this book, it would have been his seventh book in 2015. From April to July he had published two novels, a collection of poems, a collection of columns and texts from social media, a guidebook for autobiographical writing and the Finnish version of this book of Parkinson's. – *Editor*

"Weird – scientists say they have cleared the birth of the universe as close as less than a second after the big bang, before which there was nothing, because the time was born in at the same time. But the emergence of Parkinson's disease was not cleared at all so closely. Moreover, the diagnosis, the Big Bang of this condition, had been preceded even years of silent destruction in the brain, which, as we could see afterwards, had been caused a number of non-motor symptoms, so that a sensitive doctor, other healthcare professional or anyone else who could google, could have been deduced that the Parkinson's disease had started."

- At the Beginning it had Begun

- Hiding Vulnerability

"The countdown had begun."

"That's what it is the meaning of this book, to describe, what is the pain and richness of life of a person with Parkinson's."

4. At the Beginning it had Begun

There I sat, on a paper duvet on neurologist's examination table, hanged my feet like a little boy. It was autumn 2005. Neurologist – an older gentleman – had made me walk in clinic hallway, to balance on one leg, hand out my arms accordance with the instructions. He had moved my limbs, knocked on my reflexes.

Already a year or two earlier I had met occupational health doctor, but then the symptoms had been interpreted as a lack of magnesium. Now I had gone to another doctor, who had examined me more thoroughly and sent for further examination to a neurologist. And now was the time to result of the test interactions.

"It seems that you have Parkinson's disease. Have you heard of such a thing?""

I had heard, but I did not know anything about it. The only memory was that sometimes in the 80's a family friend's father had Parkinson's disease. To my mind was drawn up this friend helping her stiff father up from the chair. I had not seen this with my own eyes, I had only heard of it and captured image in my memory. Now I had the same disease. Elderly's disease. I was 48 years old. My wife was only 34, and we had a 7 years old daughter. Why was this happening to us?

Suddenly I felt like I was in the middle of American movie where the criteria for living swerve off the rails. As if I rose while still sitting towards the ceiling and looked at myself from the outside. It happened to me, but I was that poor guy who was sitting in the doctor's office and heard, that he had a progressive incurable disease. Movement disorders. Degenerative disease of the brain.

I do not exactly remember and I do not know how to distinguish what the neurologist said at that moment, what he told me later and what I read from the booklet which he gave me.

I do remember that I left the doctor simultaneously in the feelings of speedy actions and I couldn't care less. I rushed out and remained not to hold the door open for a lady coming in, as I would have normally done. I had just received a death sentence.

The countdown had begun.

Weird – scientists said they had cleared the birth of the universe as close as less than a second after the Big Bang, before which there was nothing, because the time was born in at the same time. But the emergence of Parkinson's disease was not cleared at all so closely. Moreover, the diagnosis, the Big Bang of this condition, had been preceded even years of silent destruction in the brain, which, as we could afterwards see, had been caused a number of non-motor symptoms, so that a sensitive doctor, other healthcare professional or anyone else who could google, could have been deduced that the Parkinson's disease had started.

At home I was still energetic. I told my wife contrived calm, that I had Parkinson's disease. It explained the strange symptoms. The left hand did not work properly; it was powerless and it trembled in the morning, when I woke up and turned off beeping alarm clock.

I borrowed from the library a personal book of neurologist **Kari Aho**, titled *Parkinson's as a Travel Partner* (2000). I read it immediately from cover to cover.

I studied my disease, I learned new vocabulary.

- Dopamine and levodopa.
- Tremor or trembling.
- Rigidity, or muscle stiffness.
- Hypokinesia, or slowness or lack of movements.
- Hypomimia or low facial expressions.
- Fluctuations.
- On-Off phenomenon
- Freezing.

I didn't cry until a couple of days had passed. I had just started autumn holiday, so I had time to acquire and internalize information about my illness. I called the health phone and ripped my situation.

"Do I dare to continue, do I dare to tell all? Well, I take the risk"

5. Hiding Vulnerability

After the autumn break, I returned to work, but told nobody of Parkinson's disease suspicions. In my mind smoldered hope that everything was due to the fact that the left shoulder had once dislocated. The whole thing would be mistake, a huge misconception that would be resolved. I was frightened for nothing.

The diagnosis was confirmed when brain MRI was found no tumors. "Healthy brain," the neurologist said, and for a moment I was inspired for that the Parkinson's disease was a false assumption. But the results supported the diagnosis. And in particular the medical treatment's efficacy supported the diagnosis. I felt that my condition improved considerably. I put outstanding issues in order. I was visibly eager to do things I didn't do before. I bought a new washing machine tower to replace the broken one. I was not so tired anymore. I started at work to wear a suit and tie, even if our fashion statements were informal. I built an armor of my habitus, under which I hid my vulnerability.

From all of this has now gone many years, ten years. Shock went off in time. My co-workers found out about my illness, and within a year I was already externally changed so much that easy disguise would not be successful at all. The vocabulary of Parkinson's has become familiar through experience, part of everyday life. The diagnosis was not a death sentence, but the name for a cluster of my symptoms.

I no longer feel an American movie hero lost his rails, but the star of my own life. I have to take account Parkinson's disease in my daily life with the obligations, constraints and opportunities brought by it. That's what is the meaning of this book, to describe, what is the pain and richness of life of a person with Parkinson's.

- Healthy Man among Sick

- Let's Laugh at this Disease!

"I found many people with Parkinson's to be funny, humorous and brave in the middle of their pain and suffer."

6. Healthy Man among Sick

The neurologist advised me, me – a healthy man, to participate a course for newly diagnosed. In the autumn 2006 became a year of diagnosis. It was time to take seriously my condition. I had pretty much denied the whole disease and concentrated on my job. So, I travelled by train to Joensuu, a city in Eastern Finland, famous for violent skin heads who were harassing ethnical minorities, pizza restaurant owners and alike, but also ordinary people. An old lady was beaten by a young man early in the morning at bus stop during my visit in Joensuu. The eight day course took place in a rehabilitation center, which had fitness gym, exercise gym, lecture halls, swimming pool, sauna and a lobby bar for late night conversations.

I shook hand with the other attendants, my suit jacket buttoned, tie tightly around the neck, and tie pin in a straight. They thought I was a lecturer. I did not resent it. I was pretty much myself in my work clothes and work role, I enjoyed being me. During the introduction round I told that I was working full time at the University of Helsinki as a planning officer and an adult trainer, especially as a teacher of creative writing – and I was going to do that still for many years.

I watched at and listened to the people of my group of nine men and three women. The crowd was in better condition than I had expected. If you didn't pay attention that the right hand of a gray haired man was shaking and trembling as if he were a baker spreading powder sugar over a cup cake. And if you didn't mind, that other man, younger than me, stared blank as if someone had just hit him with plank in the head. Third man was speaking as if he had swollen a rusty hinge. The fourth was stiff as fixed salted Boris Yeltsin. The fifth was holding his hand slightly bent, fingers turned in the same way as mine.

The more I learned to know them, the more I was wondering, what was the reason that so very few of those no longer were at work – unlike me, who was a slave. As the course progressed, the disabilities and preoccupations of each of us came out. At one point I was hit by envy. Why others are already so advanced in Parkinson's noble skills! They have more experience, more symptoms, more medication... As the course progressed, also the human personality in each of us was drawn up. It covered many times the symptoms of the disease. Weak voice was suddenly clear, bearing, and the gray haired man handsome, when he told us the story he loved. The expressionless face came to life at the peaks of the story.

Do I dare to continue, do I dare to tell all? Well, I take the risk. While snoring roommate kept me awake at nights, I concentrated almost continuous learning so effectively, that the various symptoms of others started to cling to me like burdocks grabbing a sleeve. I couldn't resist a deformation, metamorphosis. One night I imitated everyone in the lobby bar. This happened in a nearly endless stand up show, where I changed my voice and topics of speech to become all of them one after another. Of course my memory was laughing at me – I mixed features of several persons and created a series of Frankenstein's monsters, not caricatures as I intended.

Creepy... Was this adaptation?

- This that my thinking began to be full of holes, memory full of gray areas.
- This that my voice began to fade away, my arms and legs began to shake in the middle of the day.
- This that my findings of the social environment and interpretations of it began to be so quirky that eventually I realized I was going to psychosis.

Was this what I was preparing for myself? Yes! First, the Sick Man Role, then the Great Life Change. At the end of a hard course I was totally learned Parkinson's patient. With teddy bear pin on coat collar I send home a message: "Here comes back a sick man." I ordered a time to occupational health doctor and started directly a sick leave. I now had a new role to play, and in that role did not fit that kind of working I was used to. If I were to return work, I no longer would accept hard working in the cost of my healthy.

The main thing – at least more important than working hard – is to nurture your health, give time to yourself and your family, and thus keep symptoms under control, so that your life is going as well as possible. Something like this I was thinking. I had now tuned to use many means. Ball gymnastics. Board games. Contacts with friends. Face gymnastics. Ice skating. Nordic walking. Outdoor activities. Stick gymnastics. Stretching. Vocal exercises.

I did not practice everything all the time but something sometimes. It was certainly better than nothing never!

We wrote a poem in Joensuu. Here is mine.

Life is hands full of troubles, but one thing ease you always: reading a good book.

It is true, that your friends can leave you, but a fantastic story newer leaves you once you have hidden it in your heart.

Today's love is dead tomorrow, but you don't notice it. The end of novel you do.

Even if I don't have any inspiration to work, love, take care of my home, I always have an inspiration to read, if not fluently then one word at a moment, then another.

Reading is a gift that benefits those who come after me.

As I read I'm here and I'm there, here in my room or at a park, and there in another worlds of possibilities and circumstances, various times from past to future.

The state of reading is holy, it is blood and flesh, it is steel and sweat, it is bread and wine, it is Golgotha and Mecca.

Use your ability to read!

Reading is a joy! Reading is a pleasure that can't be achieved by other means.

Everyone knows that the word was at the beginning, but you should also know, that at the end there is the word. Life is between those, my life, and your life, valuable, unique.

7. Let's Laugh at this Disease!

After coming home from Joensuu, after acting like maniac, which I was, after waiting so long that I could again behave myself with people, concentrate to things that were present, I began to feel myself better – yet I was still very energetic and innovative. Anyway, after all that I called Mrs. **Arja Pasila**, the head editor of Parkinson Post magazine, the voice of the Finnish Parkinson's Disease Association, and agreed of writing Style Exercises, a column which would consist of prose of mine and of poetry of **HiasTimo** (SlowTimo), my new friend from Joensuu course. We started at the beginning of 2007, and wrote in each number for three years.

To be honest, I found many people with Parkins on's to be so funny, humorous and brave in the middle of their pain and suffer, that it seemed to me obvious that the style and point of view of my columns would be comical, ironic, laughing – in the spirit of bad jokes: "I'm not crying. I'm only dying." So, read ahead and make up your own mind, if my columns are funny, or at least entertaining, not only ridiculous.

"Although Parkinson's disease is said to maintain your appearance as young, when face does not wrinkle, we embody the impression of age also in other ways. The step is shortened. The hand is closed. Facial expressions have been reduced. The movements are slowed down. When eating, food drops to your trousers. All this is something else than a young man's actions."

- *Positive Changes*
- *Young Again*
- *Whales and Dolphins*

"Young. Younger... Uh! It should be enough that one gets diagnosis under the age of fifty. It really should. Why must we pretend at this age that we are still young?"

8. Positive Changes

fter obtaining a diagnosis of Parkinson's, so many positive changes have occurred in my life that it's hard to believe. I am proceeding mainly forwards, not backwards – or, not all the time backwards.

First, the uncertainty has vanished. A vague symptom cluster without the name was a heavy burden to carry.

Now that the uncertainty and vagueness have left my life, I have much calmer state of mind. If new wacky symptoms occur, I can now site them in the classification of diseases.

Mimicking a deli ad: "A good diagnosis, a better mood."

Second, medication, self-care and lazing have improved my ability to cope. Medications and exercise produce good feelings, so does lazy lying on the bed, say, with a book somewhere near and eyes shut or open. I've always been lazy exerciser and I move still too little, but for me it has been important, that after the exercise session I feel physically livelier, more powerful and more able to do this and that.

Thirdly – and this is the most important thing – now it has become clear to me the secret of my beauty and youthfulness. While the fifty years mark line was coming nearer, I wondered, why I'm in the mirror same young man as ever. And even more I wondered why people tended to call me "boy" more often than I would like to listen.

Now I know that Parkinson's disease maintain a youthful appearance, at least, look alike young. Peers become wrinkled as raisins, dried grapes. But I will tread the Earth's crust as a baby-faced boy! What does matter the fact that my brain degenerate, as long as I look, smell and taste fresh.

I look forward to my Parkinson's progressing, so that all these three change factors develop favorably. The mind is better day by day, year by year, my body is spryer, and when the boy is getting more handsome the more the peers are getting ugly.

Maybe I could say something humorous in this late night show of us. How about the idea that a young man with Parkinson's, a man like me, can experience the life of an elderly person in due time, the youngest albeit decaying cerebral. So he is ahead of his time.

Didn't laugh? At all?? Serious??? OK. Me neither.

9. Young Again

Parkinson's disease includes experientially paradoxes, contradictions, peculiarities, which I do not really want to get a grip. But I try anyway, or what you say.

Think for example the fact that in Parkinson's field we are used to call people with Parkinson's under 55 (or 50, it depends who is talking) years of age as "young persons". Furthermore, we think that those who are diagnosed under 62 years of age, which is the average onset of the disease, are "younger diagnosed than at normal age".

Young. Younger... Uh! It should be enough that one gets diagnosis under the age of fifty. It really should. Why must we pretend at this age that we are still young?

The truth is that at least I was already preparing for the role of an aging gentleman, when I got the "youth" back – unsolicited and surprisingly.

I've already managed to become a grandfather, but still I should be able to think at least another five years, that I am a young, young grandpa!

Although Parkinson's disease is said to maintain your appearance as young, when face does not wrinkle, we embody the impression of age also in other ways. The step is shortened. The hand is closed. Facial expressions have been reduced. The movements are slowed down.

When eating, food drops to your trousers. All this is something else than a young man's actions.

The paradox arises, now I realize it, because on the other hand I've got diagnosis younger than is the average age, and, on the other hand, because the variety of symptoms make me look older than those at the same age.

So, in relation to the other in same trap I'm young, but in other circles, for example, in a canteen or with grandchildren, I am or at least I can feel old.

10. Whales and Dolphins

had not made a trip abroad for approximately twenty years, and I had already deceived the idea that I would not do that in this life. I had last visited Estonia, Sweden and Mallorca in the 1980s.

I had no passport, no identity card and no international payment card, because I did not need them. In Finland I came along with my debit card and an old cardboard driving license.

After Parkinson's diagnosis my thinking changed. Life and functional capacity limitations appeared to me differently than when I was so called healthy. If I was still going to travel in more or less good condition, it had to be done now!

In summer 2007, I went with my family for my 50th birthday celebration to the Azores. The Azores is an archipelago belonging to Portugal in the Atlantic, around 1 500 kilometers west of Portugal. The island group consists of nine islands. Our trip went to the main island San Miguel, the capital city Ponta Delgada.

The trip went well and routines handled in no trouble. What's going on in a hotel room we were wondering when the lights were not working. I didn't realize that the key card should to be put atrial wall socket, and so electric was working. Well, this thing cleared out in the hotel's reception desk. However, the episode reflects the fact that the world of travelling was a big stranger to me.

43

What experiences of the trip I still live in my mind?

Ponta Delgada and the surrounding villages with narrow streets, still narrower stone ornament sidewalks, one way streets and cars speeding like mads. Gardens with flowers, palm trees and other green trees. Houses of lava stone, ceramic tile decorations. Illuminated buildings in the evening darkness, music, cafes.

Tour to the Crater Lake was the only single rainy day, which was a shame. The mountain was covered with clouds, and a beautiful lake was slept under the fog only in our imagination, not on seeing.

Fish Dishes! They must be mentioned. We ate every dinner at a different restaurant, and invariably meals were delicious - swordfish, tuna, shark, octopus and best of all Swedes served at their restaurant the fish of the day, which name was never discovered. Fish of the day was even better with "sweet potatoes" – sweet they really were, and only later we got the idea that we had eaten – sweet potatoes!

On my birthday, July the eight 2007, I took my family to dolphin and whale excursion. I wanted to remember the 50th anniversary at the day when we were sailing on Atlantic all together with my wife and daughter and whales and dolphins.

11. Elephant's Memoirs

As far as I remember, our topic now is the ability **to** remember. Memory is one of the most fundamental human and elephant properties, it's something that makes us human (or elephants).

Elephant has a proboscis with which it can miraculously pick up even a needle in a haystack, but man has a shorter beak, so we have to use hands to search for the needle. In this case, care should be taken that the needle doesn't inject – it is, as you feel if you touch it, sharp, which no doubt you knew. In the event of an accident, the injection hurts, and it may be the last straw that breaks the camel's back.

Our topic, as we all remember, was at this time, if I remember correctly, the prospects for the future, which is the opposite of memory. This is related to the saying that one does not see beyond his nose, which, I hope, you all agree. An elephant has to take a look further than a camel, if it wishes to see beyond the proboscis, which is due to the fact that the camel has not proboscis but rather long neck. For this reminds me very remarkable case, when the Helsinki Zoo camel bite a donkey or was it a mule. Life in the zoo is not the ever-blissful lounging in the sun, but, for example, monkeys can make an irritating noise.

A monkey, as you must have heard but not believed, is a close relative of the human, which have often poor postural – this is remarkable if you look open eyes – and all this monkey talking since Darwin has modified us alike the orangutan gorilla chimpanzee baboon sloth, although science has shown that baboon sloth is not monkey (neither human, even though it sometimes feels like it). So, what I had to say? Exactly! In many modern family the roles of father and mother are mixed, with the result that the kids get confused, because the differences between the father and mother is visible only on Saturday evening in the sauna. Even then the peace of hot air may hinder the eternal and unending arguing of the question if Dad promised to take the kids to the circus, a zoo or an amusement park:

"But you promised!"

"Did I?"

"You promised you promised. Don't you remember it now?"

"I remember."

"What do you remember?"

"That I promised."

"But do you remember what you promised?"

"No... Did I promise something?"

- *Move!*
- *Everyday Top Moments*
- *Out!*

"You must keep the focus on walking so that you don't fall."

12. Move!

Motionless mover has been left to my mind from the studies of philosophy as a young man. I wonder what it was and I wonder who wrote of it? Some sort of a deity, as I recall, the principle behind all, the root cause and a goal, and the one who said so was Aristotle.

I personally feel I'm often a "motionless mover", because I'm doing things of all kinds in my mind, but I do not very much like to move exercise. The tackiness of starting has destroyed many intentions to go, say, for a walk or a bike ride. Beautiful days have streamed past when looking the dirty window glasses.

However, a good mind has been the reward those times when I have gone and moved. Walking and bike tours by the river or in the nearby woods or low rise area have given numerous life-giving observations and experiences. By following nature I have been able to schedule myself and my life a calendar — I've seen budding signs of spring, felt the first frosty morning bite, heard the nightingale's song.

As I write this my head warms, but once a week warms up my whole body. On Tuesdays, namely, I play floorball. I started this sport last fall. From the previous play in 1977 was the 30th anniversary. Running behind the ball makes me sweat comfortably, legs and hands and heart get work. Learning the rules and possibilities of the game also feeds the brain, new skills spirit my mind. The sauna after the game is crowning the pleasure.

After this annealing I must make a confession. I don't fail only to do my outdoor exercises properly but also fail in gymnastics and stretching. I know that I should, and every day, but for some strange reason, I don't manage to include them in the program of my day. I remember every day to read a journal, as well as to drink coffee, but I have not created as natural routine for a daily gymnastic exercise. As if avoiding these activities could make me forget that I have Parkinson's disease.

It has not helped that the sloth make me ashamed. It has not helped that my wife complains my saggy belly. It has not helped that my neurologist has said that Parkinson's disease in combination with obesity and inactivity is a bad equation. Moving due the illness is itself difficult, but being overweight makes it even more difficult and repugnant, which of course in turn increase the kilos. Terrible vicious circle! My neurologist said I need to eat only half of what I currently eat, so I could lose weight and waist circumference decreases. Movement is then easier.

Despite the psychological resistance of my emotional level my intellect pious hope is that I achieve further development of the "movable mover", to become a mover of me on a daily basis.

13. Everyday Top Moments

The top moments of life are, after all, only a few. Thus, a good mind must mostly tear from everyday life.

Many of the little everyday doings grow to big issues which need extra power. This is a fact to people with Parkinson's. For me, cutting the pizza is a hell on Earth. Sweat runs down my forehead when my clumsy left hand tries with a fork to hold in place a pizza skating along plate and the right hand with a knife tries to cut it into pieces. Sometimes I have said that this is my last pizza.

How about the buttons of shirts and underpants? It takes time when the thick badge rolls near the lips of the hole. Often I go underpants buttons open. Almost always I have remembered to close the zipper.

Writing is slow, while all the time I have to correct hits and swings. One word takes a long time, writing one page is eternity. That's why I write now briefly.

You must keep the focus on walking so that you don't fall. When you are applying stability you are slowing down, so that the grandmothers are faster than you.

Fortunately, sometimes when you are rested enough and you do not feel the thrill because the medication is right, you are eating, dressing, writing and walking almost normally. You don't always even remember how you have suffered, when your fingers are not convulsing, your hand do not tremble nor your foot is stiff. In this case, everyday life is more or less the feast.

Good life, physical and mental succeeding in a satisfying way on the trick on the track of life produces well if not a better mind.

14. Out!

I came out to the public with my Parkinson's not only in magazines of Parkinson's organizations but also in my books few years after diagnosis.

More widely I came out as a person with Parkinson's in an interview of *Helsingin Sanomat*, the main newspaper in Finland, just before Christmas 2008. The article told that in spite of Parkinson's I had still enough imagination and that I had published three books in eight months.

From this story our neighbors, the residents of our house and many other people got to know my illness. Some reminded me of that, even years later.

One man said that it is terrible to see how a human being is destroyed like that. It wasn't very nice statement, or? I think he said too much. I wondered it for a long period. He was a lawyer, maybe that explains his rude words, but it shouldn't.

The interviewer was a journalist and writer **Taina Latvala**, who later published a novel, where journalist Latvala is remembering, that she had gone to do a story of a person with Parkinson's without knowing anything about it.

"Once a co-worker offered to cut chicken in pieces, when I tore it with fork to bite-size."

- Towards a Better life
- I'm Not My Body
- I Now Turn in My Bed

"Relationship with own body is one of the trickiest."

15.   Towards a Better Life

Not satisfied with my physical state I started to change in the multidisciplinary process of improving the life, lasting for six months.

These I want to change:

- Health (Parkinson's disease, mood)
- Exercise (bad condition)
- Nutrition (overeating)
- Excess weight (I weigh 100 kg)
- Snoring (seismic)
- Relationship (tested)
- Social life (scarce)
- Work (meaningfulness decreased)
- Writing (compulsive target?)
- Mental narrowing (empty life)

I started to write a diary, which I mark the actions and feelings related to the change. Writing is not only to document the change, it is also including motivation for change: I want to write a story of success! The diary also provides a forum to reflect and to question the phenomena related to the change and my own behavior.

I discuss, for example, what is the change for the better. It is something that the desired mode is desired, more or less different from the present. Circumstances can change, but is the aware changes of human possible? If so, to what extent?

Can a person just like that decide to begin to live better, despite the constraints? Yes! My life changes. I will change. In this way I have the courage to think in order to get the necessary kick to change and motivation to go through the hard process.

The amendment also raises the fear and resistance. How easy it would be to stay in a familiar and safe! This I recognize in myself. If you want a better life, overcome your fears, track down your internal resistance!

16. I'm Not My Body

What is my image of my body? Is it the same as my body? No, it is not.

In my mind I am young, slim, and spry. Therefore, looking at the mirror amazes me. I don't recognize the man, who has huge stomach sack.

Relationship with own body is one of the trickiest. On the other hand your body is familiar. You can feel it all the time with its pains, tremors and rigidities. On the other hand, it is like a foreign object, in which you are attached involuntarily. Some kind of alien!

One would think that taking care of own body should be close to everyone's heart. Still, I neglect my body, I think it is the home of my clear mind. I take my body as the same unconcern as a child, when healthy exercise was everyday playing, running, climbing, skiing and tobogganing.

Trembling body is crippled. I must admit, when I this time look at face of the truth. I'm crippled, lame, fall into disrepair. But in the hurry of everyday life I do not remember this, and that's good. It is a kind of mercy to oneself that the body image is better looking than the more and more damaged body.

"Once a coworker offered to cleave chicken breast, when I tear the chunks with a fork."

17. I Now Turn in My Bed

Hear – I can again in the night turn in the bed. Oh, that feels sweet! Makes a wonderful mind turn the flank just for joy. Relish the fact that I can.

About half a year, I could not. In winter and spring, my condition deteriorated throughout the period. Became more functional limitations. I had to rise halfway to sit, and even that was not easy at first. When sitting I had to change the focus to the other side and then tumble back down.

Also some other things became difficult. A fork and knife for eating was no longer successful. I ate alone with a fork in the right hand.

Once a coworker offered to cleave chicken breast, when I tear the chunks with a fork.

How about something as simple as dragging trousers?

It was not at all simple!

Simultaneously with the physical functioning the mood began to weaken. Symptoms of depression were clear. Working was unpleasant. Students also found out that something was wrong. In team meeting I told supervisor that I'm falling apart, both physically and mentally. I thought that the time had come to stop work. When the idea was clear, I got to my head in despair that the family shall go the same road. I would move to live alone.

Fortunately, I met occupational health care before I did anything precipitous. The occupational physician sent me to investigations to a neurologist and a psychiatrist. I got a chance to discuss my problems. The Parkinson's medicine dosage doubled during the summer.

The living improved. I could use a knife again and pants rose briskly. And at night I was able to turn over and fall asleep again immediately without disturbance.

Future expectations were clear again. Surely I could live with my family. The work would endure to at least one year. When the summer passed, and medication had been the right position, the mind already began to ripen for several years of working. I started happy to take levodopa, the most important Parkinson's drug.

As a young, healthy, without understanding I thought that drugs are toxins, without which I would have to live.

As an old, sick and wise I delight in each pill, which gives me a chance to live like a human life.

- At Work with Parkinson's
- One Man Team
- Have I been Left Alone?
- Whirlwind
- Neuropsychological Test
- Towards the End of the Year
- How to Survive November
- Socially Active Year

"All is well as long as I maintain the strength that I have now."

18. At Work with Parkinson's

In 2010 I was on the front of a dilemma, which would become crucial important to me at least next five years. But let's go back spring 2010 and those thoughts I had to think and those decisions I had to make.

What kind of blog should I write in this website called Parkinson's Place? It wouldn't take long to tell my symptoms; and I have talked about them enough in the columns I wrote to Parkinson Post magazine from 2007 to 2009. I'm looking forward a new point of view.

Blogging itself is familiar to me from the beginning of last autumn, when I started the Palmenia Writing Program Blog at the University of Helsinki. It is part of my job, although my topics are also such as my role as a writer and the way I'm writing.

Maybe I could write here episodes from the life of employee who suffers the condition. I happened to see, that the website called in English something like "As good as the disease can be"(awkward!) handles in next number the issue of people with Parkinson's at work.

This is for myself right now a topical issue because the Parkinson's Disease Society of Southern Finland had a couple of weeks ago a meeting for people at working age here in Helsinki. We decided to meet regularly in the future.

The Regional Secretary **Soile Kauppi** gave me an idea to found a Facebook group for the needs of our group and for the national connecting and discussion of people with Parkinson's at working age, and there has already been discussion started in a small but growing group. The group is secret, visible only to members.

I would like to tell you, now at the beginning, something about my situation at work. I work as a planning officer and a teacher of writing in Palmenia Writing Program at the University of Helsinki.

I got the diagnosis 2005 and I stayed in a partial disability pension 2008, when I started to get tired too much. By the summer of 2009, my personal resources waned, and I thought that now is the work of Montonen done. But it wasn't! Last fall I first doubled up Sifrol and then started Sinemet (levodopa), which boosted me feel better, so that now I feel again that I'm working well.

As there is highlighted in the discussion forum, writing with keyboard has become increasingly difficult. This is tiring, because my work is mostly writing. And at home I should be able to write those books I've planned...

19. One Man Team

I **wondered my job** at the weekend. At this moment I work in a "team", where I am the only member. A colleague of mine is at the alternation leave. Although we do not do the same work then, when he is here, after all he is a team member, a divider of plans and ideas.

So I am the only one who is responsible for ensuring that work is done. There is of course my boss (also known as "superior" and "manager"), but she does not participate in the practical works. The responsibility weighs every day, and it makes the work challenging and interesting. This responsibility is also associated with some kind of feeling of power: I do all the time independent decisions.

All is well as long as I maintain the strength that I have now. With my ten years' experience and routine a normal day rolls at work.

But when the symptoms are tormenting more, the lonely responsibility engaged with the power feels a burden. In my mind I keep on talking that there should be a co-worker handing out jobs. It should be so that we could smoothly do each other's works on holidays and sick leave. If we were two, the volume of operations could be increased. Now when I make about 60% of the working time, activity cannot be increased.

I talked to my manager an initial bit of this today. I have to remind the manager of this item again later, otherwise nothing happens

"Have I too early become a member of the community of people with Parkinson's?"

20.   Have I been Left Alone?

I **wrote recently** that I had talked to the manager of my thoughts to get a colleague to share my work and to develop and expand our business. I would like to continue to work as long as possible, despite Parkinson's, but now I have the feeling that it is time to share responsibility with another specialist to secure the educational process.

In order to put my intentions into practice, I sent the suggestion via email to my boss. She shared my concern that I do not have deputies in the event of incapacity for work or rehabilitation, and said that when a couple of the unsolved matters becomes clearer in May and June, we will return to this issue.

That answer was bothering me. I felt that I did not quite become heard. As if my cause, and my concern would be secondary, subordinate to some of the problems of others. When they will be solved, let's see what is left for me.

This feeling was in addition to the fact that I had already earlier felt that I had been left alone to handle my field. I like the independence of work, but sometimes it horrifies how much of it rests on my broken health. Perhaps the organization is just waiting, that I break totally and the Writing Program can be stopped. Such paranoia I developed at weekend! Today I loosened the pressure by sending our correspondence to the director and the administrative manager. I thought that it is a good idea that they know what the situation is. I didn't want that my worries and plans are only a discussion between the manager and me.

I look forward to what happens next. Probably they offer me for part-time help some employer who have spare time but not the expertise of my field and no innovative views – and which is more harm than useful to my daily routine.

21. Whirlwind

The occupational physician sent me due to new symptoms to a neurologist for consultation. The experience was as if I had been in a whirlwind.

"Now we start to treat this disease!" neurologist declared. During the next hour it became clear that she was the actual personality, exuberant storyteller, performer who spoke seriously. She even cursed couple of times in the middle of the huge stock of anecdotes. I wondered whether she had all the moving elements in right places in her head.

After studying my symptoms and medication the neurologist said that I had "a number too small medication." She made changes to my levodopa treatment. Sinemet out, Stalevo in! Stalevo has one more ingredient, it should make me feel better. For a period of generic substitution I got a sick leave. The control visit is in two weeks, just before the start of my vacation.

In addition, she sent me to three hours neuropsychological tests to assess my ability to work. I once have done that, hopefully this is a different and more demanding, and would test more broadly. After the test, the neurologist will evaluate whether I'm still capable to working life.

I also got an advice to go to physical therapy, and after that, I heard, I would be "a new boy". By the neurologist my neck and shoulders and back muscles are blocked from lactic acid.

Somewhere in between, she told porridge recipe.

I had expected that this would be as understated neurologist reception as that which I had used to visit. "You're now he," I said at the beginning of the visit. But she was quite something else, the real image of herself.

I felt unreal, when I returned to work. It felt good, that the neurologist was dedicating my particular situation so thoroughly, but on the other hand bad, as if I were sicker than I had willed to admit.

All my activities were an effort to cover consciousness of inevitable, gradual destruction. The end of life would not be living but taking care of the disease.

Now, when I write this, I know that this is too dramatically expressed. But because of I'm writing, we know that something important has moved inside of me, dragging step by step towards the meeting of reality.

22. Neuropsychological Test

Before the summer vacation I was in neuropsychological test. I got a written statement of the results and after the holiday we talked about it with my neurologist. Some of the functions exceeded expectations, in some cases there was inertia and viscosity and, for example, memory distortions with regard to details.

The statement suggested a number of measures to be done, of which some has been already implemented. The neurologist summarized as a concluded that I am able to work for years to come.

I was delighted. Like a weight had fallen from the shoulders. During the summer break I had in fact already matured a bit on the idea that if I would in the near future or immediately leave the work. I have a tendency to fly with fantasies, and I imagined myself already as an active retired. Well, a neurologist returned the realities of the place by saying I'm fit for work.

I am very much confused about these conflicting pressures: healthy versus disabled; work versus a disability pension. It seems like a self-portrait and identity would be blurred. They would gain nourishment of whom I am dealing with. For example, Parkinson Place, at least I feel in some way I belong to the great sick and retired ranks, but when I left the neurologist I belonged again to even greater group of working people.

Have I too early become a member of the community of people with Parkinson's? The neurologist advised me to consider retirement after several years. She asked about my family situation, and when I told that we have a 12 year old daughter and my wife is younger than 40 years, she said that so much is still pending. I understood it myself. Afterwards I decided that I do no longer "enthusiast" so much Parkinson's disease and related ancillary actions but to concentrate on other aspects of life.

23.   Towards the End of the Year

Hello, my blog! And hello you all, fabulous readers! A joke. What you say? There is no readers, not a single one? Bloody hell! Whom I'm writing for? And why? It's been a while since I've been writing here, I know, too long, perhaps... Over a month!

So, what's happened in the meantime? There is really no gripping to tell but something after all...

- I feel smoother after the summer's medicine changes.

- I've been writing and editing the booklet for person with Parkinson's who is still working.

- I've worked immersed in the marketing the writing courses which starts this autumn, teaching and designing a new short story course. I am no longer considering retirement, but the expansion of our team and our operations.

- Facebook group of people with Parkinson's at working age has delivered experiences, and even new members have become more and more, but there is still accommodate up!

- We have gathered once in Helsinki with the working age group of the Parkinson's association of Southern Finland, discussed together and made the Parkinson's and labor guide booklet; text version is already well advanced. The next meeting is scheduled for next week.

- I wrote to the magazine of Finnish Parkinson's Association a story of our Helsinki group and the leaflet offense.

- At home, we had the Rest of the Summer Festivities with few friends and relatives. I stayed up half to eleven, although lumbago had struck a couple of days earlier which made me tired.

- The younger daughter started middle school.

- I'm working on a novel manuscript, which will be completed sometimes near or distant future.

- I have withdrawn my participation in Tuorla meeting. Trips and happenings and jobs had accumulated too much for August. I also needed distance to my suddenly increased Parkinson activities.

- There was not room enough for me in Kankaanpää Tyyne course.

- I started physiotherapy in health center's mixed group. The private sector's individual physiotherapy was too expensive for me.

- I bought with a grant a new laptop and a printer. This is the first day I'm working with my new "typewriter".

To summarize: the work, family and situation of living have calmed near to normal. No great emotions. No doing this and that without sense. No endless reflections, to be or not to be at work.

Life is now. Not excellent, but sufficiently satisfactory. And when you know that the worse is to become, not immediately but one day, you actually enjoy the time you have now when you can.

"Outside paid employment there has been two interesting opening, which are at least temporarily boosting the view. Both request is associated with Parkinson's activity, that is, there seems to be more voluntary work. I have begun to value the Parkinson's related jobs more challenging and rewarding than paid work, which I have done by the same employer for more than ten years. When the work is typified, by volunteering I can open new visions."

24. How to Survive November

Working at the dark autumn... I remember how 20 years ago, in the fall, I started as a teacher of college, where students not only studied but also lived from Monday to Friday. The writing program was called, believe or not, Dante Academy, and no imagination is required to understand that it was a writing school with high standards. It was cited in the middle of farms and fields in Kokemäki, in the western part of southern Finland, near Pori, the famous Jazz City.

Older teachers said that precautionary to November was wise, because November is dark and gloomy and the students' ability to cope has been put to the test. We decided to organize banquets and other activities to stimulate the students live through November.

I've got the rush of this autumn eased when at the end of October ended a course at which I taught. I should have to take a vacation immediately after the end of the course, because of fatigue and lapses, which conquered my mind as soon as the effort was over. I said few days ago to the manager that physically I feel like coming to work, but mentally it is more difficult. The work seems right now rehearse the old, it's repetitive, there is not correct spark and enthusiasm. Some days working has felt disgusting, wearisome, a waste of time.

Getting a pair to work with me has after all progressed slightly. Now my boss is ready to propose to the management that it would be recruited a part time or half time planning officer; I do, as you may know, less than 60 % of working time. Together, we would be about one full time and full headed employee. The aim is to ensure the quality and scope of the activities of Palmenia Writing Program, to make possible the development of the program as well as to guarantee the continuity of the whole brand, if and when, in the coming years, I retire on disability pension. Those kinds of grounds I wrote to my boss.

The fact that I wasn't very much happy about this turn of events, describes the moods of depression of mine. On the one hand I felt relief and mild enthusiasm that I can transfer my skills to another person, a potential successor. On the other hand there awoke feelings of abandonment and surrender. What if I feel myself a vanity, when someone healthy makes my former jobs and I find out that I no longer have any meaning at work?

The supervisor asked me to describe the future of our duties; I'm going to maintain myself important tasks, so that previous vision of threats is not the only one possible future. Change can also be bracing, when we get to our routines some new blood, new ideas and new points of view. Perhaps two persons sharing responsibilities helps me again work motivated in full strength.

Outside paid employment there has been two interesting opening which are at least temporarily boosting the view. Both request is associated with

Parkinson's activity, that is, there seems to be more voluntary work. I have begun to value the Parkinson's related jobs more challenging and rewarding than paid work, which I have done by the same employer for more than ten years. When the work is typified, by volunteering I can open new visions.

That's the holy day of moods and conclusions.

I started with my memories, I will end as well. In my youth The Saints' Day, or All Souls' Day, marked working, because my mother and my grandmother were flower merchants. I have spent many of these days at cemetery gate area selling wreaths and twigs. Also, Christmas, Easter and Mother's Day marked the merciless working, no rest and peace. Now mom and dad have been retired for many years, and today when I went to say hello to them, I took three major festive yellow chrysanthemum branch. "How did you know that just those I wanted!?" mother exclaimed. Good mood came over me.

The success of my experience of the peer support group encouraged me to participate in a meeting of people at working age with Parkinson's disease. It was organized by the regional worker of Finnish Parkinson's Association. The threshold to participate in this event was already much lower than the peer group."

25. Socially Active Year

The year 2010 has been a year of social activity. My social circle has expanded. There are also new born connections of old friends. I have attended many events where I had before imagined it's not for me. How could this happen to me, although I am socially reclusive type, and my tendency for that has only accentuated while Parkinson's disease progresses?

In the first half of year I felt myself lonely. Due to my partial pension working time was only 21 hours per week. After paid work and housework there was still plenty of free time, part of which was spent to my literary hobbies. But writing was also very lonely. I began to want in addition to co-workers and relatives other chatting companies. I noticed that outside work I actively contacted only a couple of my closest relatives. Local Parkinson's club was not for me; I had not been able to go there. After I became aware of the problem, I wrote it in my diary, which certainly was the first step to solving this problem.

My wife had for some time been a member of social media called Facebook. I followed in a bit irritated mood, how she discussed with acquaintances, including my adult daughter with children's. It was ironic, that news came into my ears via Facebook faster than directly from the mouth of my daughter. Sometimes my wife showed me photos and video clips of these little girls in colorful Facebook sides.

I felt bitterness mixed with envy. Never would I want to participate in that kind of a fad than Facebook! I opposed the participation by instinct being not able to rationally justify it even to myself. Maybe I was afraid. What? That it would become visible how empty and boring I was?

However, one of my coworkers attracted me to join Facebook. It had unpredictable consequences. My need for social participation erupted in the spring as a tidal wave. Facebook made it easy to bind again relationships with friends over the years. The exchange of news and chatting became a natural part of everyday life. The online communication also led to other activities: for example, I began to have lunch with the son of my brother. The life and children of my older daughter became much closer when I was able to keep track of their doings via my daughter's status updates.

Social network increased opening up the courage to take the next step. I noticed in the Parkkis magazine of the Parkinson's Association of Southern Finland that the association organized a peer support group for sufferers of Parkinson's disease. I connected the office and asked, if I can come along, even if it was already more than four years from the diagnosis. Sure you can, I got the answer, if you feel the need to peer support group.

I went, even scared, and I did not regret it! During the five gatherings I got several new relationships with other person with Parkinson's. Later in the spring I wrote to Parkkis magazine an article, entitled "For me opened up a new world" to describe my experience in peer support group.

The success of my experience of the peer support group encouraged me to participate in a meeting of people at working age with Parkinson's disease. It was organized by the regional worker of Finnish Parkinson Association. The threshold to participate in this event was already much lower than the peer group.

At April's meeting we agreed that we would continue the meetings. It gave birth to the working age group of Helsinki area, and it has acted strongly now more than half a year. In addition to monthly meetings, we have written and edited the leaflet "Parkinson goes to work", which is supposed to appear in 2011. We set up a Facebook group for communication among the working-age people in various parts of Finland.

In my view, the usefulness of social media was changed to such an extent that I decided to visit other forums related to the Parkinson's disease. The liveliest proved to be the Parkinson Place I started to write a blog about Parkinson's at work. I also participated in the conversation on the online forum of Finnish Parkinson Association of. The conversation has led to new acquaintances both in Parkinson Place and the forum of Parkinson's Association. Some of them are also my contacts in Facebook.

Little by little I found myself doing voluntary work in the Parkinson Association of Southern Finland. I work as a contact person of working age group, I made the new website of association, I spoke at the University Hospital in an information occasion for recently diagnosed. I also went to Metropolia (polytechnic school) to tell the physiotherapy students of everyday life with Parkinson's disease. My activity led to new responsibilities. I was elected to the Board of Directors of PASF and a representative of annual meeting of the Finnish Parkinson Association, which will bring more activities and social contacts.

I have been active also as a writer. In December appeared my latest book, The Author's Book, an extended version of an originally three years ago published book, which among other things includes now the style exercises I wrote to the magazine of FPA from 2007 to 2009. The book right now is a great cause for rejoicing: it celebrates my twenty years as a writing teacher and my ten years as the founder and leader of Palmenia Writing Program.

Furthermore, I'm finishing my next novel. I have done a lot of work with it during the Christmas holiday weeks, enjoying the solitude of isolation.

Rich life has its time to each tasks: lonely creative hours of work and contacts with friends.

2011

- Still Waiting
- Colleague
- What Are We?
- Super Week
- A Guide Booklet
- Parkinson's Allows Me to Work
- A Project Idea
- Welcome to EPDA Family
- A Successful Autumn

"I watched them chatting something I really didn't care about, but at some point I noticed that they were whispering and laughing in a nasty tone. The boy sitting next to me turned to glance at me and burst out laughing again. Cold awareness rose from the bench along my backbones to my consciousness: they laughed at me. They laughed at it, how I looked."

26. Still Waiting

It was really tough to go back to work after two weeks Christmas vacation in January 2011! In the evening of first working day I fell asleep at eight o'clock, sitting on the sofa!

I wrote two months ago, in early November, that the supervisor should be submitted by the management of part-time work pair hiring me. I understand that the situation is unchanged. Her presentation is not yet made, but she has promised to do it now, in start of the year. She wants according her own words take care of recruiting properly. Why not.

When a case is prolonged and jobs are done, one starts, of course, to think that is it really a work mate that is needed. Sure these works would be done by oneself just like before.

But then I have to remind myself that in addition to the rotation of the routine we must have the resources to development and expansion activities. I'm partly retired and I've got only 21 hour working week. It is obvious that this is a challenging task. And when the stress from time to time strikes, the whole Writing Program is dependent on one man. It's a bad thing, and if there would be some catastrophe with my condition, it would be a sad thing for all of us, both me and my students.

So I'm waiting peacefully the new workmate... Maybe he or she is hired before the power completely runs out of me.

Or at the latest at the time.

27. Colleague

About a year ago I wrote in my blog that I had spoken to my manager of my wish to get another planning officer and teacher of writing to my mate in Palmenia Writing Program.

This spring the goal is realized. In February we started the selection process, and a little dragging on for a long selection process is now over. New work mate will start work in mid-May.

I know that I can get him a good and reliable coworker. I'm done with him co-operation for 15 years in two different training organizations. He is familiar with our practice.

How do I feel now?

I feel tired. The selection process was experiencing, we had several good candidates. Yet I feel also satisfied, calm. I am preparing for the fact that I need to be able at the same time to rotate our activities normally and to familiarize the newcomer with his duties. This is done before the summer recess. After the summer holidays we have a team co-operating.

I feel that some particular things have helped me to keep my working place pending the receipt of the idea of working pair

- My membership in Parkinson Place.

- Facebook group of working age people with Parkinson's.

- Writing and editing the booklet of Parkinson's for employees and employers.

So thank you all, who have read my pondering here, and supported the work to cope with!

Now I can, in good conscience, to seek even rehabilitation measure. There are about to begin in the autumn two courses involved those at work. I thought apply again. Since the autumn, there should be time and mental capacity to learn new quirks.

28.   What Are We?

Because of Parkinson's I go, on Tuesdays, to physiotherapy organized by health center. It's a functional group, which oldest members could be my parents. Usually I have felt myself in this gang as a Superman. But last time I made a mistake. I started to exercise in front of a mirror. In the mirror I saw a creature, stiff, slow and expressionless. Is it that what others see? Am I to other people an old man, who affects to be emerged from Moomin comic or escaped from hippopotamus documentary? Is it that, who I am?

I tell you this not because I want to torture myself again and again, but because I wonder: what I felt to be me, was a different person than the one in the mirror and thus the one other people supposedly always saw. This phenomenon is perhaps ordinary, universal and human, but was I really not aware of the second I?

Parkinson's disease causes changes in the appearance. Facial expressions and gestures are reduced. Stiffness and clumsiness increase. Tremors, convulsions and involuntary movements conspicuous. Not everyone has all the symptoms, but most of you may know Parkinson patients the disease will appear. However, I was pretty well rejected the idea that one's own condition yet to appear. Besides, one can get used to own symptoms so that they are just not payed attention. I was also accustomed to the fact that the left arm was bent and the hand is often compressed into a fist. Sometimes I had seen my reflection in window or similar, but only momentarily, so the picture I had fantasied to myself was not broken. When I moved out in front of the mirror, I was at the same time moved to the familiar image of myself.

Sometimes other people act as a mirror for us and gnaw self-image, for example, spiky comments. It can be thoughtlessness or cruel honesty. Last Sunday, for me, something happened, which paved the way for reflection of my few days later exercise.

I sat at the back of the bus in my own peace in a way to say hello to my parents. Three or four boys came to bus and sat near me. One of the boys was sitting next to me, bulky and arrogant, back me up, feet in the corridor, and the other sat around him. I watched them chatting something I really didn't care about, but at some point I noticed that they were whispering and laughing in a nasty tone. The boy sitting next to me turned to glance at me and burst out laughing again. Cold awareness rose from the bench along my backbones to my consciousness: they laughed at me. They laughed at it, how I looked.

I stared in front of me, I was like I did not understand anything, and I cling to the possibility that I had interpreted the situation incorrectly, that they were laughing at someone else. But at the same time I knew that this was not the case. In my mind I tried to make up them words, speech, explanation that it had said to me already before that my face looked like Groucho Marx and that I had Parkinson's disease and that is why I am such an eyes wide looking guy. When the boys went off the bus, one of them glanced at me timidly. I was hoping that he would see me as something else as subject of laughing.

The entire rest of the day and the next day went by intellectual work when I tried to convince myself that all other people did not consider me ridiculous looking. And even if they did, I'm a lot more, a lot more valuable and more meaningful. I had to lift to my mind my efforts and achievements in studies and at work, and in the written field. I had to remind myself of the importance I have in my family and social networks. I had to revive the trampled human dignity of mine.

Self-image is changing slowly, but now it's as if it had become destroyed in a single bus journey. To some extent, I was still the blond-haired, skinny fast feet fox that I had been forty years ago. I was unaware that my hair had darkened over the decades, now grizzled, that my step had been shortened and that ribs would no longer be visible, if I came towards camera chest naked as seen in the 1970s film. I had known all this, but I cherished deep down the image of myself as a young man, even though I was of course connected to the pile of self-portraits, which I later in my life had drawn to myself to the chambers of my mind. At the age of fifty+ I was of course already working on new pictures of myself, but only slowly and gradually they were moving to self-image, which most strongly I felt to be my own.

Now, suddenly a lot of me died there on a bus bench. I'll never be the same. Always I would be a ridiculously looking man, suspicion does not disappear ever again. Thus, when on Tuesday at exercise I looked at the strange object in the mirror, I finally did not at all stop at the idea, that is this the way others see me even though I feel different. Somewhat unwillingly describing aloud to the physiotherapist the image in the mirror, I was wondering the possibility that I myself would be that strange object, stiff, slow and expressionless. Maybe I was even hoping that she would deny, but she just looked at me with sadness in her eyes, as is looked the one who tells the truth.

29. Super Week

Sometimes the occurrence condense, are packed so close together that the impressions are subsequently almost impossible to see one at a time, separately from each other. For me, this was the Parkinson's Week, which was celebrated this year, 2011, from April 11 to April 17, just after the parliamentary election campaign culminated before Election Day.

Actually, I took a head start for Parkinson's already the previous week on Friday, when I talked about "Working with Parkinson's Patients as a Challenges of Everyday Life" at SoveLi Fair in Helsinki Metropolia University of Applied Sciences.

Speech and a PowerPoint presentation lasted only twenty-eight minutes, but the mental preparation took several days. A little shaking and voice-colored I pulled performance through without any effort of stage charisma.

What challenges has an employee with Parkinson's disease? What must be taken into account in order to toil at work and still have energy left for free time? When is it time to leave the job and get a disability pension?

I got the diagnosis of Parkinsonian the middle of the finest working life, 48 years of age. The neurologist said or partially asked that you still want to do a bit of work. Now "a bit" has continued for five and a half years, and is still going on. I have experienced working so important to myself and for my wellbeing that I want to keep on working as long as I can.

Work is not a number of dice, but to approach the issue of the challenges of Parkinson's patients at working age, I'm imagining this dice by all sides of the cube describing a different challenge.

1. The adequacy of the medication is the first challenge. It is the basis of continuing at work and coping with it. The finding of right medication ensures that the health status is stable enough to make work possible. I go regularly as well as occupational health doctor and a neurologist to make medications to keep up to date. After all, a progressive disease is in question.

2. Exercise, maintaining physical fitness, is another important challenge. After diagnosis I exorcised diligently according to my neurologist's instructions, but at some point self-motivated exercise and stretching stayed. Now I take care of my physical condition in a physiotherapy functional group organized by the health center. We meet on a weekly basis. Between the meetings I'm riding at home my exercise bike and practice gymnastics stick. I have still much to do with my physical raising.

3. The third challenge is to continue full time work, or possible transfer of part-time work. You have to take account both remaining resources and economic considerations. My solution was to remain partial disability pension three years after diagnosis. Short working hours and enough leisure time help to cope and revive at work. All the time I need remains for the

Parkinson's activities, volunteer work and social recreation.

4. The fourth challenge is to ensure that the work is still fit for you. All former tasks may no longer be suitable because of increasing amount of symptoms. In particular, the tasks needing strength and dexterity are not suitable for a person with Parkinson's. Can you choose the tasks? Are some of the tasks wasting of time and easily dropped off? In fact, I chose my favorite tasks, when I stayed at partial disability pension. The most stressful tasks were transferred to another employee.

5. The functionality of the working community is the fifth challenge. I understand that a good and open relationship with my manager and co-workers is important. It is an advantage if they know that my strength is limited, the fluctuations of my endurance and ability to work, and weakened ability to cope with stress. The workplace must also be able to react to my changing needs. Recently my role has expanded and the pile of tasks has grown so much, that it has become topical to hire me part-time colleague to share my work.

6. The sixth challenge is the mental ability to cope. At work I have to avoid stress and pressure of timetables of concurrent multiple tasks. For this occupational physician has properly written an opinion to my employer. Emotional coping is helped, if you can maintain a good mood, positive attitude, in spite of an incurable progressive illness. Emotional coping is threatened, if you feel you are disabled, freak, and odd. I have found peer support people of working age to help with these feelings.

I am working as an expert on the computer. Tremor, rigidity and slowness are not an absolute barrier to my working. In contrast, when mental well-being and curiosity threaten to end, it's time to move to entirely disability pension

.

30. A Guide Booklet

Just in time before the Parkinson Week appeared a booklet "Parkinson comes to work." It is a voluntary work force sample. The idea was born right in the beginning of our group, in the first meeting, when we were defining our purpose, tasks and targets. We decided to do something useful for the benefit of society. Soon it was clear that we would do a guidance for employees and employers. I informed the Finnish Parkinson Disease Association, which took the booklet in its program. **Mr. Tapani Mauranen** wrote and edited the text with me. I delivered the idea and draft in social media in order to get assistance. Dozens of Parkinson patients participated and put forward new ideas of the content, made suggestions of editing the text, either directly, or making proposals, and also by telling stories.

The Parkinson Association of Southern Finland organized four thematic happenings during the Parkinson week. I informed of them with the help of local early morning radio. I myself attended the first event, when I visited Monday afternoon Kamppi service center gymnasium and played some ball games. I had wanted to go there to play already before this occasion, but now under the banner of the theme event I succeeded. It was pleasant to meet fellows from East of Helsinki and from Espoo, the next city West of Helsinki.

On Tuesday, my intention was to participate in the Finnish Parkinson Foundation seminar in Biomedicum at the University of Helsinki , but after a half working day and physiotherapy functional group I was so tired that I stayed at home. Later, I heard that there had been about 350 people, and no more would have fit. All the material that the Parkinson Association of Southern Finland had reserved had run out.

On Wednesday, I met a group of people at working age in the office PASF. The first hour we spent in discussion and planning of future activities, during the second hour I told about writing a life story. We had a little reminiscence exercise. At the end of the hour came up an idea that I should organize a writing course to the members of our association. It starts at the beginning of October. New members have joined our group of people at working age along the way so much that mailing list has already about thirty names.

On Thursday I attended a Parkinson activity only online via Internet at Parkinson Place and the Facebook group of people at working age. My writing in *Helsingin Sanomat* had collected feedback comments in these forums from different parts of Finland, which pleased me.

On Friday, I went to Joensuu, where was held the 10 years anniversary of Parkinson Association of Joensuu. I met many acquaintances, some of which I knew already only by the net, and got to know new acquaintances. I participated the meeting of the working age population committee where we went through the experience of actual operations and planned the future.

On Saturday it was held spring meeting of Finnish Parkinson Disease Association in Joensuu. I was now for the first time a union representative giving my input at the national level for the affairs of the Finnish Parkinson Association. There was an important proposal to be decided concerning the future of an old school estate, which was used as an action center. It was an economical burden to the FPDA. After many questions, memoirs, opinions and other speeches I realized, that nobody had said yes nor no of the proposal to donate the school to separate association, which would take care of the activities and economy. The chairman said that one more comment, and I used it saying yes for the proposal. The gavel hit the table. Resolution was adopted, as no one had objected it.

Parkinson week was followed by a torment week, super week by a super fatigue. On Monday, I nearly fell asleep at work. The idea did not move. With big difficulties I got something meaningful done. My mind tried to work out the last week experiences. What was the significance of the events? I could not get a grip on. Best thing to do was to sleep overnight.

When on Tuesday I was coming back home after a six o'clock from the board meeting PASF, I had the insight of something. It was a warm, sunny evening, and in the gentle light I saw my Parkinson activity from a broader perspective.

I understood that important Parkinson contacts to me was also a large number outside the local group and association. There were already dozens of friends, acquaintances and business partners all over Finland. My reference group was nationwide. I understood that local activity was important, but a fruitful co-operation and supporting of community were not limited to the local.

So, I realized that during the Parkinson week my inclusion was strengthened to the entire Finnish Parkinson community from north to south, from west to east. I was grateful for that. The next step would be the internationalization.

31. Parkinson's Allows Me to Work

The shock is like a sudden death, when among the best years in working life the neurologist gives you a diagnosis of Parkinson's disease. For me this happened five years ago. I was 48.

The shock was not any reduction in the acquisition of basic knowledge about this incurable, progressive brain damaging disease and movement disorder illness, which main symptoms I had in my own body: shaking or tremor, muscle stiffness and slowness of movement.

The diagnosis is always a shock not only to patients themselves but also to whole affected family, spouse and children. So it was with us.

What kind of life there is in future, when one of the support pillars of family has long term illness? Perhaps sooner than you can imagine he or she is unable to work and needs assistance?

Spouse easily meets the worries and fears. Is there a pressure, that you must forget your own career and start to think yourself as a caregiver? Everyone is not ready for that.

Illness of an employee naturally at least raises questions among employer and workplace. How long the employee can continue to work? Is a person designated as key worker still reliable team member? Should we already start to look for a successor?

After the initial shock a disease is adapted, including Parkinson's disease. Adaptation represents a realistic image forming of one's own resources, possibilities and future.

Also in the workplace happens adaptation, especially when the employee is able to continue. All are not able to. Much depends on the nature and severity of the work, whether the work, for example, needs physical strength or is demanding dexterity, so that it is poorly suited for Parkinson's disease for. Around half of those affected in working age is retired full timely within two years of diagnosis.

By various means the career may be extended if the employee's physical and mental condition are good enough and she or he has a desire to continue working. One way is half time pension, which I have chosen. At the same time when my working hours have been reduced, workload has decreased. I have left out tasks that pose the greatest haste and stress. This requires the employer sympathy.

Occupational Health Physician follows my condition and coping with work regularly. I turn to a neurologist when I feel the symptoms increased and my medication is in need of revision.

Coping at work will also facilitated by peer support, sharing problems and joy with those who are in same situation. Across the Finland, in such cities as Turku, Helsinki and Rovaniemi, people with Parkinson have begun to organize themselves in peer groups and keep in touch with each other. Peer support can also be given online, for example, Facebook, which has its own group of people at working age with Parkinson's disease. Facebook group does not know of localities and the land borders.

After obtaining a diagnosis the future pictures of normal life were dashed. In their place I imagined, though unwillingly, images of rickety, drooling human ruin with tremor and uncontrolled movement. The career in working life would be over during next few years. Horror images have not been realized in five years. Instead, I have learned to take the future more confident and calmer. The disease progress slowly, so I have time to adapt to the inevitable changes.

Parkinson's disease has not prevented my working, it has rather made the job more important factor which gives me the daily rhythm and meaning.

Helsingin Sanomat 11.4.2011

"I learned a lot in a short time. And I have again noticed, what kind of power has a human, who may work in the mode of excitement, with the object of own interest and for the benefit of important matter."

32. A Project Idea

The last week of May was so busy that I have seldom lived through such a week. In addition to my own work I wrote a grant application to RAY (*Raha-automaattiyhdistys,* Slot Machine Association) for an important and interesting project. The project is called "Parkinson's at Work", and as you can see from the name, it is associated with activities of those who have got Parkinson's disease diagnosis in working age.

The week was very intense. I used almost all my free time for the project plan. I worked with a group of people which included both employees of the Finnish Parkinson's Association and the volunteers with Parkinson's disease. I sent the project plan to them for comments, I made after that additions, clarifications, depreciation, and sent again a new version for review. This continued until the plan was clear and convincingly presented and justified.

Lofty aim of the two-year project is to support the welfare of people with Parkinson's disease at working age by adding the endurance at work, family and hobbies. The aim is also to extend working careers, which will benefit both employers and employees.

The concrete idea is to support and develop and gather together the activities of people with "working age by creating a web site, which is aimed at people of working age, as well as their loved ones, employers and the workplace. We have on the site news, articles, calendar of events, blogs and discussion forum. Site content is mainly public. Some of the functions need registration with a pseudonym.

The service website is maintained by the part-time project worker and a network of volunteers. The project organizes events, seminars and training related to the theme of the service site – including writing courses for bloggers.

The Finnish Parkinson's Association and the Parkinson's Association of Southern Finland do co-operate with the aims of constructing a national network and supporting local activities of working age population with Parkinson's. We hope, that the users of the new site consists a community supporting individuals, with activities also outside the network.

It is now about six months to wait, how the financing succeeds. Preliminary decisions will be made in December.

I learned a lot in a short time. And I have again noticed, what kind of power has a human, who may work in the mode of excitement, with the object of own interest and for the benefit of important matter.

33. Welcome to EPDA Family

"**Can you hear my heart beating?**" I asked the audience, who had just patted my presentation. I pressed my lips against the microphone: "Tutumk! Tutumk!"

I was in a workshop of European Parkinson's Disease Association (EPDA), the umbrella organization of numerous national associations. The workshop was held in the context of the annual meeting of EPDA near London in October 2011. Nearly hundred people from about thirty countries took part in the workshop and annual meeting. I represented the Finnish Parkinson's Association.

In the presentation I had told, how we wrote and edited, with the help of volunteers and social media, the booklet *Parkinson's comes to work*, published in the spring by the Finnish Parkinson's Association. The guide was translated into English during the summer, the translation was published just before the EPDA meeting in print and online. Prior to my performance I shared the *Parkinson's comes to work* booklets to participants in the workshop.

Our guide was well received. In particular, people liked its most eloquent style, which many considered being different from the typical publications, which aim to illustrate Parkinson's disease. I got already queries that can the text be loaned and applied to informational materials they do in their own countries.

Successful appealingly style was in great extent created by Tapani Mauranen, another supplier of the guide.

My presentation took place in the morning of our starting day. Half an hour after the start of the workshop, I had already taken care of my share, and I was able to concentrate on the rest of the program. I did not have any specific expectation, so what I got in those few days consisted partly surprising but quite interesting and useful items. In retrospect, in my mind will rise three subjects that I want to tell you.

First of all, it became clear how various European countries has diverse conditions in the treatment of Parkinson's disease and also in the resources of associations. The number of specialized neurologists and Parkinson's disease physicians varies. For example, Finland has reportedly twice in proportion to the population of neurologists compared to Sweden. Parkinson's nurses are not known everywhere.

Many Parkinson's associations struggle along without public funding; in Finland RAY finances activities. The lack of public funding means that the associations do not have paid employees but all action is dependent on volunteers.

And it was me who went suspenders pounding to tell the audience that we have made the booklet properly by volunteers...

The number of patient membership in Parkinson's associations varies. A country with populous equivalent as in Finland may have only two thousand members, when the Finnish Parkinson's Association has about eight thousand members, of which people with Parkinson's well over five thousand.

The total number of people with Parkinson's disease in Finland is estimated to be about fourteen thousand.

The workshop offered me different ways to approach the sufferers of Parkinson's disease. The Swedish representative told us that they have volunteer telephone dispatcher, to whom those who have recently received a diagnosis can call, and all the others who are in need of discussion and help. Switzerland has built strolling bus, which disseminates information and promotional materials. Other means to approach people with Parkinson's was to establish radio station and focus on social media.

Secondly, **I drew attention to the** warm atmosphere there was at the workshop and meeting. Everything was less formal than I expected. Very quickly emerged collegiate atmosphere. We worked for a common cause despite our different starting points. Group activities took place in interesting, mainly constructive discussions.

Of course, the atmosphere was also created by social events and situations, joint breakfasts, lunches, dinners, corridor discussions, line dance and rock'n roll. The exchanged business cards encourage to communication in the future.

EPDA made a deep impression on an emotional level. This experience contract summed up best the Secretary

General Lizzie Graham, who said to me: "Welcome to the EPDA family!"

She added that when we get somebody here, we try to keep him or her to come again. So I too was invited to participate the EPDA's workshop and the annual meeting next year in Amsterdam. There the weekend begins with Parkinson's Unity Walk.

The third point, which caught my attention, was the need to broaden the perspective on Parkinson's activity. In my life, I had already managed to expand my horizons just from the perspective of receiving a diagnosis to active Parkinson's patient's perspective. The meeting and group work should have been seen from point of view of Finnish Parkinson's Association and, in general, from the perspective of the situation in Finland. In this I was not always able to do my best simply due to lack of knowledge and lack of experience.

Among other things, presentation of various projects broadened to see things from European perspective. 1.2 million Parkinson's disease sufferers is already quite a large number. We heard demands such as the right to early diagnosis, the right to effective and symptomatic treatment, and the right to a qualified doctor twice a year.

And what is a global perspective in Parkinson's disease?

Parkinson's disease is estimated to be suffering from 7 to 10 million people in the world. The expansion of perspective from the individual experience to a global mindset, from the micro level to the macro level, is not quite painless process. It takes work and studying, writing and reflection, skill to dance and polite kissing, but it is also rewarding.

Excellent chance of learning provides third World Parkinson Congress, which will be held in Montreal, Canada, in 2013. It brings together scientists, neurologists, people with Parkinson's, caregivers, physiotherapists and other medical or relevant professionals. There I can surely meet the EPDA family.

"And when the stress from time to time strikes, the whole Writing Program is dependent on one man."

34. A Successful Autumn

When good things happen, you have to enjoy it. You have to stop for a moment, and really think hard that this is true, this is splendid, and this happens to me. You have all the right to congratulate yourself, because you are at the moment the Number One!

The three worlds were one. The highlight of the fall, so far, especially emotionally, was launching of my two new books in October. During the evening, the atmosphere was as if I was in a scientific discussion, going to defend my thesis, initially nervous, but towards the end of the evening I relaxed more and more. About 50 people had arrived to listen the presentation of my sixth book and third novel *Sadie Q* and my seventh book, a diary of changes, *Towards a Better Life.* Or maybe they came to listen a panel discussion, which was attended five other writers and teachers of writing. The audience was both my former and current students, few people with Parkinson's disease, colleagues, strangers, and my older brother, who said afterwards that the Parkies were a nice bunch of people. Perhaps he got rid of his prejudices.

While I presented the books I talked also about my Parkinson's disease, of which I write in the diary of changes. In this conference organized by the University of

Helsinki I wanted to reveal myself to view, including the private adversary, and do not act only as role of writer, planning officer or teacher. At speaker podium I felt myself a whole person, when I did not have to hide tremor and condition.

Literary world, the world of work and the Parkinson world met each other, were one.

In Parkinson Place there has been talking about happiness this autumn. That evening I was happy, and my satisfaction has been the main feeling in my everyday life ever since.

Oiva has born. It is a club for people with Parkinson's at working age, known earlier as a "group". Oiva is now one of the official clubs of the Parkinson's Association of Southern Finland.

By the change of the status the amount of duty bearers have increased. I am the President and Press, in addition there is now a vice chairman, the secretary, the fund manager, club manager and one person responsible for culture.

For the different projects we set up working groups. We have already a planning group, headed by the vice chairman, for the forthcoming nationwide meeting for early onset and young people with Parkinson's, including those who feel themselves young.

Operation of club constitutes of meetings monthly in the evenings at the office UPY in Helsinki, Friday cafes which are also on a monthly basis during the mornings in cozy cafés, as well as recreational trips and events. You can become a member of Oiva from the whole area of Southern Finland.

Wild joy filled me, when I heard that RAY presents a grant of EUR 60 000 for Parkinson's at Work project. The Government of Finland decides on grants finally in February, but in general, no changes is made to the presentations.

The project is as close to my heart as it can be. Hopefully it offers methods to solve problems that people with Parkinson's at working age meet at work and at home. I was diagnosed about six years ago. I remember the words of neurologist, when he had found the Parkinson's diagnosis and turned his gaze to the future: "You want to do a little work?" A little! It had gone only fifteen years from completing my studies! The major part of my career should have been in years to come.

In response to diagnosis I hung myself to my job, it became more and more significant part of my life. Sometimes too significant. I have been able to set work to a proper position only with help of partial disability pension and volunteering. There is more to live than working life offers.

But how long can I be part of the world of working? "You are still able to work for years," said the current doctor a year and a half ago. With the help of good and adequate medication I have done my job perfectly well and enjoyed working.

Parkinson's at work project is natural, almost a necessary extension to the series of actions during the last couple of

119

years. Voluntary work receives more established form of RAY's funding. The project offers more resources for information and peer support, participation and sharing of experience. The project supports both regional and national activities.

I am very glad and relieved of the decision of RAY and look forward to what the project will bring to our life. A clear mind and a big heart, an honest mind and human touch, all that is needed to the succession of the project. The project is only a tool, the content itself is more significant.

- Social Challenges
- A Strange Feeling
- Under the Surface
- The Site Opened with Manifesto
- The Last Word

"If I were truly interested in an exchange of views, I would ask questions, I would help others to talk about themselves as far as that situation would be possible."

35. Social Challenges

People are crackling. Telling but not listening, comparing news, experiences and views. Let's talk this and that. Speech is innocent, harmless, not too personal, not deep stabbing. It's a kind of talk, when relatives and friends meet at social events such as birthday parties.

Empty Head. I'm feeling as I've got an empty head. These events occurred in the summer holidays twice. Both times I made a similar observation: I have lost my ability to talk. The difficulty is not my voice, but something else. The sound I should have, but nothing to say.

I have become boring. Most of the topics of conversation do not interest me. They are frivolous to me. Some of the topics I do not understand. They are too difficult to me. Some of the topics for discussion have been scoured for years or decades ago. They are history to me.

Frivolous, tough and old topics could, of course, been talked and listened to what others have to say. Perhaps the point could postpone me more important, easier and more recent topics. This is how people act: "From that came to my mind..." And then it would be your own subject at the heart of the debate.

If I were truly interested in an exchange of views, I would ask questions, I would help others to talk about themselves as far as that situation would be possible. It would not take long when of the interlocutors would reveal interesting features, which could continue the story. People like the fact that they are listened to, that someone focuses on their world.

My problem is that I no longer get on my mind anything that I could offer for a new angle of the discussion or could attract partners to open up debate.

I don't react other people's speeches in my thoughts and I do not produce questions to hear more from others.

I have closed to myself among other people, who have wrapped up the discussions around themselves, without contact with them, and the air is filled with lines of speech.

My head is empty, empty except for the horrific feeling that I grasp myself more and more disabled by Parkinson's disease.

What if there is no correlation between Parkinson's disease and this remaining speechless, what if it is typical behavior to me. I do remember from my earlier life similar strangeness and external experience, especially among people I have not met before. But these latest muting have occurred in groups where I should feel safe and confident, where I should feel myself accepted.

Would it be a non-motor symptom, after all? My wife tells me that my behavior has changed in a few years, as the disease has progressed. It is as if some kind of surface shell of good behavior had peel off me. I'm tired of no longer in social situations to try and present as much as before. Especially now on vacation I have not only become more private but also more primitive. Others company has annoyed me, made me angry, made me recite awkward dirty words the rare cases when I have opened my mouth.

The result has been the shame and self-accusation, anxiety and depression, which at its worst, so I am afraid, can lead to fear and frustrations of new social situations. Why go to parties to suffer and swear, if I'm feeling restful at the company of my own...

It remains to be seen whether the head will fulfill of thoughts after the leave, when the work and Parkinson action begin. For the end of the summer and early autumn there will be number of trips and social events that provide opportunities to practice conversation skills.

"It's as if the brain had shrunk, as a tight circle had been round my head."

36. A Strange Feeling

What is this strange feeling, which has now continued for two days? Or was this already last week, but I did not pay attention to it, because I was, from Monday to Thursday, part of the day at work? In the workplace you somehow slip to your work role like a hand in a glove, and the strange feeling could not come to the surface. Even in the morning when you walked from the railway station to your office you strengthened yourself to your duties at work.

But yesterday, when I spent my retirement day at home, a strange feeling hit me. It's as if the brain had shrunk, as a tight circle had been round my head. The legs were powerless, muscles without arousal. The whole body was stiff and a little bit of vibration.

I sat on a chair of kitchen staring the clock. When I had last time taken the drug? How long would it be to the next tablet? I expected that I would strengthen as long as the drug would affect. The morning's first drug did not help me to the normal feeling and the ten o'clock drug brought no relief. I tried to improve my condition by relaxing in sauna.

I had promised to clean, but the plain thought seemed disgusting and too heavy. I managed to fill washing machine and dishwasher. That was something! But I could not go out to buy food.

After the two o'clock drugs I looked an hour and a quarter television, the combined ski and jumping. Sleek upstanding young men jumped on air, when I tried to jump from the couch's convenience out to the store. Afternoon blurred.

Finally, I felt myself so strong that I took my bag and left home. Fortunately it did not rain. The cool air felt good. I walked briskly across the yard and over the road to trade, I did my weekend shopping and I came back. I was the winner!

Evening was spent like so. I was inspired to write up important e-mail so surrendered that I forgot to take my evening six o'clock drug. I woke up at seven in the hand cramped and I went to the medicine cabinet. Rest of the evening went to drinking tea and watching television, at nine I fell asleep.

During the night I woke up the usual two or three times, stopped by restroom and kitchen, and got up in the early hours after four to read the paper and e-mail. I heard a nasty news. I replied sympathetically. At six o'clock I started the daily medication and began to make breakfast.

Even though it was a Saturday, I was getting ready for work, namely the voluntary work. This autumn I have taught on Saturday mornings at the Parkinson's Association of Southern Finland autobiographical writing, writing your own story. I went to the store on the way and bought coffee and something to eat and at the office arranged everything ready the pupils to come.

A while it felt like everything would be in condition, but as the day progressed, and the ten o'clock drug did not work, I felt a familiar band around the head again, I felt I'm an outsider, and I really was not able to keep such a tight schedule as the situation demanded. In the end we were half an hour over a regular time, so that all had a chance to present what they had written.

One member of the group ride me home and I took immediately afternoon medicine and warmed late lunch. Again, I had promised to use the vacuum cleaner and could have still go for shopping, but both seemed impossible. Had I not done already enough today? I postponed jobs and immersed myself in email and on Facebook, until while the afternoon dusk I rejected the trade mission as vacuuming for the day.

My wife phoned from work and asked whether the home tasks are done. I told him that I have another day feeling strange and I cannot now. What kind of feeling weird? It is difficult to explain. As a Parkinsonian. It feels like your body and mind and your muscles do not have the power and right as if you do not have brains in your head... Try to find your brains from the hangers, my wife said before she hung up the phone. She had announced she would meet her friend after the work.

Tomorrow is Sunday. Vacuum cleaner is waiting. Perhaps a visit to a shop to fulfill the refrigerator. And then comes Monday, and work day. I hope that I can once again slip into job roles and feeling as a stranger remains in the background. Familiar situations at work and well known practices support the "I", which is broken. At work I am more than a brainless muscle cramps trembling. At this illusion I want to live yet a moment.

"I used to voluntary work so much time and energy, that it was like a second job."

37. Under the Surface

Suddenly I began to feel that I was fooled, brutally exploited. My expertise was good enough, good enough yes indeed, and over a wide area. I planned, wrote and taught. Free. Why? Because I was kind. I wanted to help. To feel myself necessary. Volunteering had become equally important – no, even more important! – than wage job, which I did on part time basis. I had been at partially disability pension for four years. The two last year had been increasingly full with duties. I am employed by the Oiva club and the local and national associations. And social media. Some of the jobs were invented by me, to some were I was requested information or they came to me because of my duties. Stamina was put to the test in those days, when there was first in the afternoon the meeting of Board of Directors of our areal association, in the evening Oiva club board meeting and after that the club meeting free for all members. I used to voluntary work so much time and energy, that it was like a second job. In that sense, I would be very able to continue to work full-time. In the workplace I erected approximately the same amount of work as before full time. I worked without a break, I drank a cup of coffee at the computer and I did not sit with other employees in the coffee room answering the ten questions of a local paper. I had a lunch though. I was cheap labor. I received a salary of less than 60 % of the former. I received a disability pension of 50 % of the pension. Although these together are nearly 110 %, remaining money was hundreds of euros less than the full term. This combination worked so and so. Sometimes you had to use credit card, but the holiday money and tax returns, and other random inputs I received, were enough to get loans repaid. Until this spring, I was resorting to credit card more often. Expenses without warning. Household appliance procurement. Daughter's camp fees. Monthly subsidies paid to civil action, and the adult daughter. I realized that the economy is not working. I made hectically work from morning to night, after coming home from work I opened my laptop and I continued volunteering. I helped others, took care of others, but I could not take care of myself and my family. Then I thought that am I stupid. I let others make me idiot. Nothing should take precedence over personal and family well-being. For other should be given only an extra, be it money, time or care. Soon I would be in bankrupt, client in social office, begging in the street. I decided that change must be done. I made a plan. The idea was to focus to large entities instead of frustrating minor details. **Job:** I'll put the partial disability pension to rest until further notice and come back to full-time work. This surely makes better the economic situation of the family. **Writing:** rather than writing here and there short texts, I'll begin writing the next book. I had applied for a grant to write, but I'll finish the manuscript no matter did I get a grant or not. **Volunteering:** I'll stop working in many levels of organization and concentrate on one thing. It is enough, when I give my contribution to Parkinson's at Work project. After making these decisions living became easier, step became lighter, forces increased. I did my earlier missed household chores. I returned empty wine bottles to liquor shop, glass jars for recycling. I went to a long walk. It would start a new, responsible time of myself and my family. Happier life. Not so much sociability, but instead of it meaningful working days, monitoring and supporting the progress of the project, creating moments of a new book. Reading, remembering, thinking and writing – surrounded by the melancholic melodies of the Finnish Radio. Once the decision was made, the heaviest was done.

"The project is only a tool, the content itself is more significant."

38. The Site Opened with Manifesto

Now the Parkinson's at Work web site is complete and open for users. Together with the Project Planner Anna-Maria **Salonen** I have planned and then ordered from a visualizer and a digital media company the actual construction of the sites. Now at the start the web site has only few pages with detailed content: the first blog post, start of the debate together with notifications of few events. The web is like a cultural center or activity to which only participants bring content and creative spirit. The online service provides a framework, a playground, conversation arena for those, who are interested in the relationship of Parkinson's disease and working life.

Parkinson's at Work site's message is "Information, Support and Activities for People with Parkinson's Disease and Working Communities."

When we were planning the web site we liked to think more than just the people with Parkinson's. What does a progressive long term sickness mean in the workplace? What should supervisor and co-workers know? How collaboration can aid disincentives for Parkinson's disease sufferers to continue, the energy to work?

Among other things, these kinds of questions we hope to answer in the writings of network. We want to offer both facts and reports from lively work. The experiences shared by the users of the service are at least as valuable as statistics.

This manifesto consists of three principles on which I base my actions at work.

- A person with Parkinson's disease has the right to work for as long as he or she wants and is able to.
- The employer must support the continuation of career of person with Parkinson's by arrangements and action which make working possible.
- Working community must adapt to the changing capacities and resources of a person with Parkinson's disease.

39. The Last Word

I f in the beginning was the Word, from which all was born, is there a word to which all ends at the very end? What is the last word? And who says it?

These questions I have pondered from time to time when the debate on Internet forums has accelerated and the issue has begun to bother outside of the network in everyday jobs, hobbies and family activities. At best, the debate is leading a lively sparkle of intelligence and brain gymnastics, the use of the word feast and rhetoric joy of playing. In spite of the body solidifying illness the word has been alive!

But at its worst debate is endless repeating the same stupid arguments instead of factual argumentation. I must admit that I myself have succumbed to a bad debate culture, I have become angry too easily. I have done far too fantastic interpretations. Little Devil has come out of me. In part, the reason may be personality characteristics, in part all the changes brought by the disease experiencing and thinking.

Online conversations, like other fighting, have a cycle of life. Start can be mild or shocking, carefully prepared or full of surprises. Docile start can soon lead to arrogant sequel, when someone on the line has different opinions and shouts out his or her own controversial views. Pens and swords are sharpened, opinions are hardened to steel and speech held alternately to attack, alternately to defense. Verbal battle of high wattage flames some time and finally slows down when the ardor wears itself out.

When the fighters already a bit embarrassed in mind are collecting loose arms and legs and pieces of swords and arrows from the battlefield, in the air there is hovering the question of who has the final word, who will give the final death blow to the discussion. Requires patience, restraint and wisdom not to respond once again. Sometimes it requires the use of external mediators, in order to bring to an end the debate a decent way. In the end, pardon the silence that shelters can patch up their mind, and kicked black and blue self-image. Pain combined with their own shame a debate on how low. Recovery takes time. But a good start can be reached as to recognize that the doctoral candidate and their perceptions might be, after all, more common than separating. Follow cautious reconciliation gestures. Sophisticated courtesy. The respect. Man seeing the differences of opinion and conditions. This is my last word.

- Do Continue Working
- Parkinson's Patient in Media
- I'm Proud of Parkinson's
- Project Events
- Parkinson's in Mind
- Selective Culture of Termination
- Dreams Come True
- Empower to Dance!
- Can Science Support the Hope?
- The Most Important in WPC2013
- Local and National Meeting
- Garbage
- To Envy, Hate and Isolate

"But our speed will slow down as time goes by, the symptoms worsen and medication causes side effects increasingly. We soon no longer are sexy interviewees in media."

40. Do Continue Working

The second week in January I met a neurologist, who considered important that I'll continue in my work. The medication was changed so that in the morning and during the day I take the drugs more frequent pace, per night less. Thus medication is most effective when I'm at work.

A visit to a neurologist and his message delighted me. I got confirmation of what I feel and what I think. Working keeps me alert and in motion. As a result, I can maintain social contacts and networks.

Although I'm released from the office after 4 hours and 12 minutes, the day's work is not at the end. After lunch, I use time to volunteering, to the national Parkinson's at Work Project and to the working age people club Oiva at Southern Finland. Both live in an active phase. Organized by the project, there will be a Seminar on Parkinson's Disease and Working Life in March in Helsinki. The seminar is open to all and free of charge. In April, the project organizes in Turku a working age action weekend, "With New Strength to Working Week". In May we have a two day writing course for bloggers in Helsinki.

In Oiva club, we have monthly meetings, but that is not all. We also have bowling always odd weeks on Thursday night. Bowling is fun together when you know how to enjoy the game and also enjoy the succeeding of your friends. For May we are planning to visit Kotka, a city with a harbor in the Eastern Finland, Oiva as a guest of local Parkinson's club.

The third area I'm working is writing a novel. I started by brainstorming and writing early last spring, but the speed of writing has accelerated markedly during the current situation and rhythm at work. It has become a habit that I work with the manuscript on a daily basis. When I made the long days, I got too tired to write in the evening.

Some of my voluntary tasks ended when the year changed, necessary, which has brought more time, especially for writing. I have deliberately sought a balance between work and family life. At this rhythm I continue towards the spring and summer.

41. Parkinson's Patient in Media

What positive people with Parkinson's talk about life, when interviewed by the media?

A typical format is such a thing, that in spite of Parkinson's disease the patient in focus does something heart's content. I myself told in an interview of *Helsingin Sanomat* in 2008, that in spite of Parkinson's disease I had published three books in a short period of time. Another says that she moves with passion, gymnastics, bowling, playing, cycling, running, and ski two thousand kilometers of winter. The third travels frequently abroad. The idea is that Parkinson's disease does not prevent us from doing what we would do- without the disease. Unspoken hope is that I'm like a healthy, normal person: treat me as such!

A nother frequently seen form is an argument that only due to the disease interviewee is doing something new. Parkinson's disease get the interviewee to paint icons. To sing karaoke. To write poems. To build, to weave. Whatever. The disease is somehow activated unused regions of a person, a burst of creativity. This causes mixed feelings: you enjoy a new hobby, you develop yourself in practicing it, but the diagnosis of Parkinson's disease is hard price of the joy.

The third formula of telling life with Parkinson's is praising the new friendships and bless of volunteering. Friends in same condition are important, they are like family members, gang that understands without words. Hard work in benefit of the supporting group, local club or areal association gives satisfaction, especially if the fulltime work has already been left behind. It is a huge and wistful to think that without having an incurable disease one would not be familiar to all of the wonderful people who come to the most varied professions and from different parts of country.

The fourth story line goes so that Parkinson's disease has helped me to find my true values, to glorify my position and mission in the world, to understand the meaning of life. Enlightenment moment: I found the Story of Life. Despite the Parkinson's disease we have, at least when we are well medicated, an adorable strength to mess around, but only a limited time.

But our speed will slow down as time goes by, the symptoms worsen and medication causes side effects increasingly. We soon no longer are sexy interviewees in media.

But anyway, we left behind four beautiful stories, isn't that something?

42. I'm Proud of Parkinson's

My attitude towards Parkinson's has changed in several occasions during the nearly eight years that have passed since the diagnosis. And no doubt in the future my attitude will change more and more as the disease progresses.

Initially, after getting a diagnosis, my mind occupied consternation and horror. The sad fate was drawn up when I received the first information about the disease and its symptoms, leaflet, internet, books. Life was extinguished light. Drape yourself in the mantle of shame and fear. In the workplace I was too ashamed or afraid to tell my illness. I hear someone or something say: *I have Parkinson's disease, and I hide it under a dark suit.*

A year after diagnosis the course in Joensuu escalated my mind in turmoil. Attitudes towards myself and the disease became more permissive, when I met other people with Parkinson's, both patients and caregivers. The knowledge of this disease deepened and was organized, and the severity on this condition and its impact on every day and professional were clear. Still, my relationship with living with the disease became easier to take. I embraced a forward looking, day by day mindset. *I have Parkinson's and I cope with it.*

There followed many years of Parkinson's activity. Press coverage, associations and clubs, positions of trust, web columns and posts for thesis writings. The medication was added from time to time in order to remain the functions at work and home. I was a tirelessly working person, although sometimes so tired that the eyes did not remain open. I had a task, which made me important. I was living the hybrid of Parkinson. I was conscious Parkinson's patient. Parkinson's disease had become the main content of my life, the descriptor of my identity. *I have Parkinson's, and I'm proud of it.*

Obviously this cannot be able to go on forever. Symptoms and signs of my condition are increasing. Sometimes I'm in solid form as salt statue, sometimes the legs are moving Elvis style. Arms and legs ache, shoulders are sore, cramps are teasing me, swallowing has become difficult. I speak at the phone with nervous voice, and turn my body strangely. I have many things indifferent, I do not care. In the evenings, the entire being is painful. The nights I sleep restlessly, often in periods of couple of hours. *I have Parkinson's, and I'm tired of it.*

But there is still much to experience. Adding medication, brain stimulation surgery, levodopa pump? If I ever go stiff, despite all the care of you sit in a wheelchair, or lay down in the bottom of the bed, I can look back on this time period in which the performance was still intact and the feeling was, after all, to endure in spite of all the troubles. I did brought-in, wrote books, I went bowling, traveled, I met friends, enrolled in a dance class, and was dating. *I have Parkinson's, and I have lived in spite of it rich life.*

43. Project Events

During the spring the Parkinson's at Work Project has organized three very different events, involving a total of about 90 people, some admittedly took part in two or even three events. Within those occurrences we have divided knowledge, practiced and tested body fitness and trained writing skills.

The long and carefully prepared Seminar on Parkinson's Disease and Working Life pulled out in March. In an auditorium in the center of Helsinki was gathered more than 40 people, mainly people of working age with Parkinson's disease but also employers and health care representatives. The subject was lit by a versatile lecture. The material received during the day can be read and printed in Parkinson's at Work site.

In April, 30 person met in Turku, West coast of Finland, in the shelter of Special Training Center of Finnish Parkinson Association from Friday to Sunday. The weekend and the program was called as With New Forces to Working Week. The program was quite physical activity oriented with ballgames, moving and dancing and walking in the rhythm of Bach, exercise in swimming pool and versatile with tests. In the evening, we practiced vocal muscles by singing karaoke.

A **two day training**, targeted to blog writers, raised the convening around fifteen students and their teachers in Helsinki early May. Mrs. Ranya Paasonen, writer and teacher of creating writing, taught the first day, the second day was on my responsibility. The program offered guidance to the attitude of a writer and to the writing means and measures. Finally, we brainstormed a continuing course for those who are already writing a blog. This will be in program in October.

P **articularly important** addition to the formal program of these events has been informal meetings and chatting, making new acquaintances and strengthening the old ones. This ancillary and maintenance of social relationships has occurred until the early hours.

P **roject events** will continue in the autumn. We have planned at least one weekend action in Espoo, the neighbor of Helsinki in the South of Finland, writing trainings for bloggers in Kuopio, eastern part of Finland, and in the isle of Hailuoto, outside of Oulu in the north of Finland as well as already mentioned the blog writers Advanced Course in Tampere.

44. Parkinson's in Mind

hen I started to find out what disease I had got, I learned that the body deteriorates, but the mind remains clear. Same said a colleague when she told about his old father with Parkinson's disease. It is a "movement disorder disease". However, the cause of symptoms is decay in the brain, it is thus also a "brain decay disease".

I experienced contradictory those names and characterizations. How come the brain degeneration does not affect the mind and thinking, cognitive ability, informational activities? It is forced to make a difference! I remember the sauna veranda of our summer cottage and I crying forehead against my father's shoulder, crying that my brain deteriorates. I saw a clear view of how I turned into fog eye nonsense speaker.

Later, I read about the cognitive changes, more broadly, the non-motor symptoms, about everything else than the body moving related symptoms. I have read and I have experienced.

Although the Parkinson's Dementia would not expect right behind the door, one and another thing provoking concern should be noted.

The following observations are based not only on my experience but also in written sources. I kind of loan my persona to illustration of this serious topic.

1. Fatigue

Forces simply run out in the middle of the day, or more exactly the evening. Thinking clots. I got to get to bed early. Some people are just leaving to lively bars, when I already have inclined my head on the pillow.

2. Forgetfulness

I forget not only the individual names and words and anniversaries but also discussion, consultation and declarations of the things. People tell me what "I know" and what I have promised. Sometimes the matter is returned to my mind thus aided, but not always. Sometimes my own speech told later to me by other people are real news.

3. Lack of Meaning

Many things no longer mean anything to me. Disaster news do not move. I do not care about the carbon footprint. In social situations I am indifferent and sink deep in myself. I don't necessarily participate at all lunch discussion with co-workers, if I listen that's good.

4. Indecision

Different solutions and alternatives sails back and forth and I connect them in real time convincing features. I rent this apartment, because it is the right size and in good location. I will not rent, web declaration was already vague, one image from the neighboring houses. I rent, however, I have just submitted a binding offer, which has a penalty of one month's rent. I do not rent, I despite the sanction, I pay what I am committed and rent a new apartment only after two months. I rent now in spite of all, I want to move in right away. And this is only one example! This happens again and again.

5. Inability Initiative

This is reflected in particular to the difficulty of initiatives of leaving and doing. If I do not have an agreed reason to go, I can stay the whole day at home, inside, even if there were the most pleasant weather. No matter whether spring, summer, autumn or winter. In the evening I read on Facebook what acquaintances have done during the day. Everything: sailed, taken care of the garden, done whatever you can imagine with their cats, dogs, hamsters, rats, horses... They have hunted, driven across Finland, travelled as vacationers in Croatia ... I have looked out the window, but I have not been unable to step out of the door.

Have I changed or have I always been like this? Are these and other symptoms slowly become with this illness or permanent traits of personality? The problem is one of the most difficult. How can I allow my thinking to discern whether Parkinson's disease changed my thinking? How can I with my sanity try to ascertain whether the disease changed my understanding? How can I understand that do I grasp things now as opposed to before the diagnosis? My mind is as well the target of observation as itself the instrument to observe.

What if I've already forgotten what I used to be before this condition? It's pretty much possible. When unpacking boxes in my new home, I opened a photo album, in which appeared playful Timo, smile on his face, beautiful boy, as some girl said. I am no longer the same, I have become alienated. But why this does not mean anything to me?

"The one who looks like the weakest link of a chain, may be, if not the strongest, but a strong enough link, the employee in right place."

45. Selective Culture of Termination

The researcher, economist **Harri Hietala** from Vates Foundation drew in his article (*Helsingin Sanomat*, 22.8.2013) attention to the anomaly that some elements in law and procedure prevent the employment of people with disabilities.

This is important. But it is also important to prevent the disabled and the chronically ill falling for no reason unemployed. Parkinson's at Work project organized a Seminar on Parkinson's and Working Life last spring and we found a selective culture of termination. Officially, the disease has not been reason of termination but strangely in co-determination negotiations, the choice falls on chronically ill person, who is still fit for work.

Employment again of chronically ill or disabled person in such a situation is difficult.

Employers should bear social responsibility and offer the disabled the opportunity to continue working with support measures where required for as long as there are disincentives. The amount of work can be adjusted, for example, by part-time work and the inability retiring.

"Careers are not becoming longer unless the diseases that force people retire are payed more attention," uttered Professor **Mika Kivimäki,** in Work, Well-Being and Wealth meeting, reported *Helsingin Sanomat* (27.8.) on the previous day. "Also the normal changes brought by age must be taken account."

Often, for example, those who have in working age got diagnosis of Parkinson's disease, are conscientious and hard-working employees. They have had to face life and time constraints, which is reflected in a serious attitude towards oneself and other people.

The one who looks like the weakest link of a chain, may be, if not the strongest, but a strong enough link, the employee in right place.

Helsingin Sanomat

46. Dreams Come True

I **found the World Parkinson Congress** in 2011, when I did a search on web for Parkinson's disease.

I was immediately inspired by the congress. As I watched the videos from performances on the previous conference held in Glasgow 2010, I knew that out there I want. Next congress, the third one, would be held in Montreal, Canada, October 2013.

The idea to departure to Montreal accompanied me these few years, until in the summer preceding the congress, it was time to start making concrete plans.

I began to inquire if someone would travel with me among people with Parkinson's I knew. Definitive, the traveling companion was found near, the 15 year old daughter was happy to join me. With one condition: if one place to visit would be teen star Justin Bieber's hometown, Stratford. It's a deal!

We decided to vacation in two days before the congress in Toronto as a base. The first day we went by minibus to Niagara Falls, and on the second day by train to Stratford. Each day trip was successful and relaxing.

O **n Tuesday, 1.10. it was time to fly** from Toronto to Montreal and stay in a hotel opposite the Congress Palace. We went to the congress palace for signing up and got necks labels, which were identified by a blue bar that we were something else than scientific participants. Congressional inaugural ceremony and reception were in the evening, during the day was held lectures Parkinson's disease for the general public.

At the opening of the congress leadership told the work required to produce the event, and gave praise to the participants. Special thanks got **Elizabeth (Eli) Pollard**, who reportedly had "made everything".

The 3334 participants of World Congress had arrived from 64 countries, so the arrangement staff and volunteers had plenty of work. The winner of Video competition was announced, the winner was the sentiment of an impressive animated film *Smaller (smaller)*, which can be viewed on YouTube, as well as many other related videos of the congress. The opening ceremony also announced the next Congress venue and the time: Portland, Oregon, United States of America 20.-23.9.2016.

On Wednesday, 2.10., the first ordinary congress day, I attended eight o'clock to poster lessons. From the poster exhibition in the exhibition hall of congress was selected for each morning three performers, who told twenty minutes about the topic to the general public. In my notebook I wrote, for example, the phrase that mild cognitive decline predicts dementia.

I fell asleep a couple of times during these poster lessons, but continued still sitting in the great hall when the actual scientific lectures began. The theme was that why and how certain nerve cells die and what it can do.

"This is war!" declared first speaker.

I listened to a lecture, and then I left to an adventure in the rest of the Congress Palace. I talked in the lobby with an English volunteer settled orange t-skirt. He thought that the scientific lectures are so difficult, that they do not give anything for the layman. He recommended leaving for a walk to French district.

However, I didn't leave to French district, but I continued wandering in a large lobby where there were standing and sitting groups here and there. I went to talk with the Canadian Mark. He wanted to tell me what he knew about Finland: Nokia, Angry Birds, and ice hockey players. The following days I noticed this same phenomena: starting a conversation was easy and the people were very friendly.

Before returning to the hotel I went to poster exhibition, which was not yet open to the public but I went in anyway. I helped an Indian man to stick a big poster to the wall. I asked him about the situation of Parkinson's patients in India. In a large population, there is of course a lot of Parkinson's patients. Parkinson's society is organized and of the forms of treatment for example brain stimulation is in use.

We went with my daughter for lunch in a modest cafeteria in a French neighborhood near our hotel. We looked in quite a few restaurants before we made our choice. After lunch we took a walk on the narrow streets lined old houses made of stone.

In the afternoon I attended the workshop, which themes were music, art, creativity, and Parkinson's disease. This workshop was one of the most memorable learning experiences during the congress. The workshop discussed, among other things, what is the role of dopamine-agonists often found in the awakening of creativity. If you have met people with Parkinson's, it's almost certain you have noticed that many people write poems, columns or short stories, paint, sing, dance – even acts on stage. And these people awakened to create arts may not have in their past history any connection to arts nor creating.

Canadian **David Simmons** said he had left agonists out because did not like the upcoming thoughts: "Do this! Do that!"

Simmonds pointed out sharply that the obsessive, desire or need to create is not the same thing as the ability to create. This phenomenon I have often come across as a writing teacher.

American **Steven Frucht** told about interesting gauge witch visual arts area. There was, for example, found that while painting fine motor skills work better than usual. One artist's complex painting style changed by Parkinson's disease completely realistic. Another artist's style changed, in turn, from realistic to impressionistic. He painted day and night until the balance of medication was right. One artist who had painted house pictures painted after installation of Deep Brain Stimulator only nude pictures.

Frucht mentioned the art clinics, and I got interested in the idea immediately. The Parkinson's Association of Southern Finland, Oiva club, and Parkinson's at Work project organized at the moment, separately, singing classes, dance classes, writing courses and drama clubs, and in the past had also provided instruction in the visual arts. Art Clinic could take the form of this activity together and increase the supply of both daytime and evening groups. And what is essential, the activities brought by art clinic would also include scientific research! It would be important to get information about the effectiveness of the Art Clinic. Effectiveness, of course, is not the same as comfort, pleasure, success and acceptance experienced by artistic people with Parkinson's. Or is it?

Art Clinic could apply for project funding, so that participation could be free of charge.

Irish **Margaret Mullarney** told inspiringly of the activities of Move4Parkinson's Foundation, which she had established. In Ireland there are about twelve thousands people with Parkinson's, roughly the same amount as in Finland, but unlike Finnish the Irish people had gathered an energetic set of twenty person, which surprised the congress guests at least twice with an engaging song "Something Inside So Strong", this too can be heard and viewed on YouTube.

Margaret Mullarney told me, when we happened to meet in the lift of our hotel, that she was pretty much alone in the previous World Congress in Glasgow in 2010. Now, she had a couple of dozen bunch with him.

Mullarney introduced the activities of Move4Parkinson's Foundation in a workshop of art and creativity. People of Foundation were easily noticed by violet colored shirts, on which was printed the spine of the main slogans: Empower, Inspire, Educate.

Mullarney presented five elements, which would help to get a view of coping with the disease. She urged to try the five way to select the most suitable for oneself. At the bottom of the prospectus of the foundation was a notice that if you intend to make changes to comply with these instructions lifestyles, you should first consult with a neurologist or other therapeutic personnel.

Here are the five elements:

1. Awareness of medication & medical assistance

2. Diet

3. Exercise

4. Emotional well-being

5. Alternative Treatments

Margaret Mullarney presented a cogent question: How can the Parkinson community prove to scientific community the effect of creating, functioning and empowerment?

She called on to become out and visible and to feel around you the hands of those who share these creative ideas.

47.   Empower to Dance!

On the second congress day I listened few morning lectures on non-motor symptoms, but the most important aspect in the visit consisted of participation in two workshops, the first dealt with means to empower and second dance and Parkinson's.

These both nourished my thoughts of art clinic, especially when at the dance workshop initially was reported of a study, which showed that a group of people with Parkinson's which danced tango maintained a diverse of motional functionalities, while in non-dancing control group, these functionalities weakened. Dancing group also added more social activeness and surely experienced a variety of spiritual pleasure.

Question of empowerment of people with Parkinson's was under consideration few times. There was even a special event dedicated to this topic. I decided to participate that already in Finland when I was planning my trip. I was entitled "The means of people with Parkinson's disease to empower".

The first speaker, Spanish **Fulvio Capitanio**, asked provocatively: "Do people with Parkinson's disease want to empower?" I wondered that myself, and I wondered the people with Parkinson's I knew, and I came to the conclusion that yes, yes, we want to empower ourselves! We want that our life has everything under control and that we are able to set and achieve goals. In spite of illness we think about the future with optimism.

Fulvio Capitanio not only asked but also answered. He presented the following list of means of empowerment:

- Take responsibility.

- Set goals.

- Collaborate.

- Understand and support.

- Stay in your decisions.

- Collect the evidence.

- Be smart user of health services.

- Stay in a safe health care environment.

Capitanio showed the road of empowerment of some individuals as a curved arrow with words from the bottom to up such as Lean, Train, Teach, Coach and Advocate. The figure initiated to consider my own steps at Parkinson work. From aid recipient I have progressed to a donor of aid, from a target of charity to a source of charity, from a student of characteristics of the disease to a teacher, coach and a supporter. This was an eye-opening moment.

Empowerment is a communal phenomenon. The last note of empowerment session was: "Helping you helps me."

Tango is a good dance for people with Parkinson's disease. That came clear as spring water in a workshop, which was called "Dance and Parkinson's disease: why and how?"

I wanted to participate this workshop, because the topic was hot in Finland. I attend this fall a dance course of Oiva club.

According to American **Gammon Earhart**, the dance is good for Parkinsonian patients, among other things, because it increases activity. And tango among other dances is especially suitable because the basic step is walking. In addition, tango is a surprising dance, which provides opportunities for improvisation.

Earhart told about a trial, where a group of people with Parkinson's dance tango in an hour twice a week. Dancers' pairs had not Parkinson's disease. All danced exporter and successor roles. Pairs were traded every 10-15 minutes. Participants were examined prior to the start of the dancing and the year after. Results were compared to a control group that did not dance tango.

Tango dancers movement functions remained and even became better, while the control group's functions deteriorated. The study monitored, for example, balance, walking, simultaneous walking and talking, hand and arm activities, as well as movement symptoms.

Tango group maintained its skills by dancing still the second year once a week, the control group did not. Dance did not active only the movement functions, but it also increased the social participation.

That is true. I noticed it soon after the congress.

"We have about three years to put together a set of participants to next Congress in Portland and develop an original message to say and show."

48. Can Science Support the Hope?

O n the third day of the congress on Friday 4.10.,
Which actually was the seventh day of the
journey, fatigue began to be felt. However, I
participated special lectures, the theme of which was a
positive life after Parkinson's diagnosis. The speakers
were "three heroes", as they were introduced. **Robin
Elliott**, an American who introduced the trio, insightfully
pointed out that early diagnosis means a long time to be
different from your own community.

First came to speak British **Alex Flynn**, who blandly listed
affect a manic doings. This hero, diagnosed at the age of
46, had run 20 marathons in 10 days, ran and walked
from London to Rome, through the American continent,
in South Africa and the Amazon. He admitted that the
drugs move him. Sometimes he was woken up to the
idea, that what the hell he is doing here, in the middle of
desert or jungle.

The other two speakers were **Sonia Mathur,** Canadian,
and American **Rich Clifford**. Mathur told about slogans
she kept important, such as "Parkinson's disease does not
define you", "Optimism is a choice" and "Pay attention to
your abilities."

Clifford, in turn, was a NASA space pilot when he got
diagnosis. He agreed with the employer, that the
diagnosis is not told in the work community. He even
made a spacewalk when he had Parkinson's disease. After

NASA, he spent 15 years at The Boeing Company. His message was: "Do not give up!"

In the evening, it was time to summarize and end the Congress. Emerged, inter alia, the idea of relationship of hope and scientific witnessing. How science can support the hope? Let's hope this means, of course, the discovery of a cure for Parkinson's disease. It was also found that the pharmaceutical scientific community understands that people with Parkinson's disease have a lot of information. That is one reason why it is great that different groups from patients to researchers get together.

49.   The Most Important in WPC2013

What was the most important in Third World Parkinson Congress? The questions below function as a repetition and a method of rise to my mind the essential of the whole week:

- The few days holiday we spent before Congress in Toronto, Niagara Falls and Stratford, teen star Justin Bieber's hometown?

- Congress opening ceremony, where the heavy workers were praised, the winner of the video competition was published, and the place and time of next Congress was announced?

- The poster exhibition, of which some exhibitors were chosen to speak in front of a large audience?

- Scientific lectures, which offered prospects of what scientists involved are working?

- The workshops, which dealt with the basic themes such as dance, art, empowerment and sexuality?

- Freeform appointments for others with Parkinson's disease during the breaks of lectures and in hotel?

- The opportunity for researchers, doctors, physiotherapists, nurses and people with Parkinson's disease to dialogue and mutual understanding?

- A summary of the events in the afternoon, which crystallized essence of each day's knowledge?

- Walks in downtown Montreal and exploring cafes and restaurants and the amazingly rapidly changing milieu, the French and the Chinese district and the region consisting of high glass and steel buildings?

- Congressional conclusion session outlining the things emerged often during the Congress, such as the importance of exercise, and it was noticed that people with Parkinson's have to be faced as a whole, not just trembling being devoid of dopamine?

These were all important, but the most important thing was that we were there. I was making true my dream, which I had cherished at least two years. I was along with my daughter a part of the world-wide Parkinson movement.

There were more than three thousand participants from 64 countries. Other Finnish besides my daughter I didn't meet, some researchers there were according to the list of posters. But I met, after all, two acquaintance from the European Parkinson's Disease Association (EPDA), the Norwegian chairman **Knut-Johan Onarheim** and the treasurer **Mariella Graziano** from Luxembourg. I had danced with Mariella unforgettably in EPDA's annual meeting in London nearby in 2011. Mariella is a physiotherapist and she knows how to take fast a slow person with Parkinson's so that it seems like a really dancing with a star. She remembered the dance and emphatically said that the most important thing in dancing is "spirit". That spirit, good spirit and atmosphere, I felt at the World Parkinson Congress.

After the Congress Eli Pollard send me a message. She had followed some time my commenting in Facebook page of the Congress. She regretted that we had not met in Congress. On the final I was definitely a few meters away from her, but I t did not come to my mind to say hello. Pollard hoped that in the future Finland would take a bigger role in the World Congress. Now, Finnish Parkinson Association was not even a partner of the Congress, unlike the Swedish, Norwegian and Danish unions. She asked, if I could do something for that.

I took Eli's concern seriously. First step would be the partnership of Finnish Parkinson's Association, second step would be raising awareness of World Parkinson Congress in Finland, and the third step would be a Finnish delegation participating next Congress.

We have about three years to put together a set of participants to next Congress in Portland and develop an original message to say and show.

"I felt that all the hard work I had done for this club was not gone in vain. I had built something important, and new faces were now building on that base."

50. Local and National Meetings

Oiva's annual meeting took place successfully yesterday evening at the office of Parkinson's Association of Southern Finland. In spite of the fact, that Oiva club is dedicated for those who are still in working life or at working age, many of us have retired for the sake of age or condition.

We sat around a long table which became crowded and someone was willingly outside in a circle, because there was exceptionally lot of participants.

The meeting elected interspersed with coffee drinking briskly The Board of Directors for the year 2014. Vice-Chairman wanted quit and her replacement was elected as new. Board of Directors was expanded with one new member, who is responsible for the program of monthly meetings.

For monthly meetings, it was agreed that each time someone or some members are responsible for executing program. This can mean, for example, the acquisition of initializer.

Fundraising was one topic on the list. It was decided to order 50 boxes (each of 1 kg) toffee, which members of the club are selling for price of EUR 20 / box. The accumulated funds are used to support courses and hobby activities.

The atmosphere at the meeting was enthusiastic and uplifting. I felt that all the hard work I had done for this club was not gone in vain. I had built something important, and new faces were now building on that base.

At the meeting of Working Age People with Parkinson's committee, I told about the annual meeting of Oiva club. This happened yesterday, Friday, in the morning here in Turku, where I am celebrating the 25 year anniversary of the local Parkinson's Association. Later, at the daytime, there was a seminar, and in the evening a programmatic party vibes with dinner.

Today, Saturday, was held the autumn meeting of Finnish Parkinson's Disease Association. Last year's decision of the similar membership fee of all associations was declared invalid.

The meeting elected Professor **Ariel Gordin** to continue the Chairman following two years. In addition, the 2014 action plan and budget were approved. The meeting was preceded by researcher **Filip Scheperjans** interesting presentation of intestinal bacteria and the emergence of Parkinson's disease. The subject was fresh and the research results have not been published yet at the time of this meeting.

51. Garbage

Did it really take place without debate? An eviction of one member of Parkinson Stop, former Parkinson Place? I cannot understand nor accept, that linking to a blog would hurt the instructions and netiquette of the site. Still, the administrator arbitrarily denied this and set punishment of dismissal. Is this supposed to be a community of the members, rather than a dictatorship? Brutality, in some people aroused admiration mixed by jokes. Shame on you! IT IS real grievance, that the administrator announces to resign those, who put to appear the blog link of a specific member, including me, because I had already once added the link, and it was deleted by the administrator. I'm not the only one who was treated like this. I am concerned, that with moralistic grounds is prevented linking to other sites. Everybody knows it is an essential act in web communication. In a free society, there must be a chance to deny, argue and correct decisions. Leaders also make mistakes. That's why we have a three tiered judicial system. It is easy in this online community to raise decisions to closer look. Each member can by own interest participate in the joint review, such as now has happened. A blind faith in the authority is not an intellectual honesty.

I received a serious warning from Parkinson Stop administrator. I was warned "from now on acting contrary to the provisions for the administrator and the rules of Parkinson Stop." The reasons were, that my disregarding of the prohibitions of administrator and disrupting comments do not belong to the forum. That was the case, I read, in my writings on conversation titled "Community or dictatorship". I received this warning upright. It is hardly previously sustained that the employee of Finnish Parkinson's Association receives a serious warning in this online community – or should I say dictatorship.

A year later I left the Parkinson Stop, for good. I copied and collected a couple of days my writings and then made end of the membership and emptied all I had created. I was going to do this for a couple of years ago, in 2012, but decided to maintain the membership as long as the Parkinson's at Work project lasted. Parkinson Place/Stop was a good information point for the activities organized in the project. My need for peer group was already taken care in the early years of my membership, from 2010 to 2011. After that it was a forum for dialogue. But nowadays there are other forums for that.

In the current Parkinson Stop I was irritated by the administrator's claims that there is no democracy, but he as the dictator decides everything. I think that kind of scenario is inappropriate. This is a web community, among sick people. Well, now I have left this behind me. I reported the conversation that I copy my texts and then I close my account. I heard, that after my departing the administrator had instructed the members for resignation in a proper way. Part of that was a rule, that if you delete your content, you cause everyone thorough injury, even to yourself. <Needless attempt to make members feel guilty. Now there appears to be 14 answer. Should check them in disguise... ;)

E nd of story. I'm not going on any longer on this subject. Enough stupidity is too much (or should I say too much stupidity is enough?) to continue discussing seriously.

"People with Parkinson's do envy, underestimate, hate, isolate, tease, lie... just like other people."

52. To Envy, Hate and Isolate

Actually, now when I've opened the waste bucket, stuck my hand to the garbage, why don't I tell one more annoying occurrence? This isn't pleasant, so I write briefly only of this one case which is embarrassing me most.

This case concerns the Parkinson's at Work project, which was hard to accept to a few people. First of all, they let me know even before the project started, that it benefits only those who are hired to work at the project.

The other complaint was that the project gives nothing new to the people concerned. On the contrary, in an absurd way they made it clear, that I with my project was taking something crucially important away from them, the complainers!

And what was it? It was a concept they had created years ago to organize a local club of people with Parkinson's at working age. They didn't realize, that much had happened during those years which had passed from the start of their own club. And furthermore, the project was national, not only local, and it aimed to give support to local clubs in all parts of Finland.

People with Parkinson's do envy, underestimate, hate, isolate, tease, lie... just like other people. We are not clean as just washed plate, but most of us are not either dirty ashtray. Some of us are.

"My first book, by the way, was published in 1984, when, so to speak, I was a man with good health, although very problematic. I imagined that I was a great writer, and it was very important to me. Now I know I am, but it doesn't matter anymore."

2014

- Interviews
- 444
- All Kinds of Things Happen

"Now with PD I have a purpose."

53. Interviews

Parkinson's at Work project came to an end, but website of the same name continues to live on a voluntary basis. I will continue to do the tasks of administrator.

The web service is still a forum of information to employees and employers. Bloggers write reports of work and life. Forum provides support and interaction.

We do not organize weekend meetings or other events, at least not as often as during the project, but active blog writers have decided to gather together in March 2014 at Finnish Parkinson Association 30th anniversary on a cruise from Turku, former capital of Finland, to Stockholm, the capital of Sweden, and back. I hope the specific local working age or young onset clubs and groups continue to tell about their activities on the website.

Project Planner Anna-Maria Salonen has wrote, visualized and made the layout of final report of our project. It's quite impressive, I have to say. Thanks so far to all participants!

My eighth book, which have a provocative name, in English *I have Parkinson's, and I'm proud of it*, was published in February 2014 at Oiva Restaurant in Kallio, for me a memorable district North of

Helsinki City. Fifty or sixty people, relatives, co-workers, Parkinson's comrades, our union representatives, were bringing warmth and good atmosphere in the evening.

The book consists of 30 stories I have written to the Wearing Off website, and 13 stories from other websites. One of the writings was published in the newspaper *Helsingin Sanomat*. These 44 independent writings are in chronological order trying to create something new, now when they are together, at least experiences of a person with Parkinson's disease from autumn 2005 to autumn 2013.

I have received a laudatory book reviews and reader feedback faster and more than usual. The book has clearly a task which it fulfills successfully. It feels good when a reader shake hand to give thanks, and with the other hand shows how the tears are dropping while reading. And this reader was a man. I have also given two magazine interviews, which are not yet appeared, as I write this.

My first book, by the way, was published in 1984, when, so to speak, I was a man with good health, although very problematic. I imagined that I was a great writer, and it was very important to me. Now I know I am, but it doesn't matter anymore.

Senior Health Journal 2/2014 contains a three-page interview of my case, written by freelance journalist **Marjo-Kaisu Niinikoski**. Her story follows the story of my book. I could actually read the interview only once, very quickly.

Apu magazine (4/3/2014) has a four-page interview of my life and the most recent book. Journalist **Maarit Vuoristo** wanted to tell my story, and I think she succeeded very well. In addition to the interview, the story includes fact boxes.

Photographer **Kirsi Tuura** took pictures of me from the front, back, and side probably an hour in many places. It was real work when I had to stand with knees bent against a wall, so that I would be at suitable height for her.

I gave one more interview months later, in October, to a family magazine *Seura*, quite similar as *Apu* is. The interview appeared at last February 2015. Jounalist **Mari Kaukonen** writes as part of my story also about my mental problems, pychoses and depression. These are nothing unusual to a person with Parkinson's. Photographer **Mirva Kokko** managed to snatch the picture just when I looked an Old Man!

"Cranston lifted up as the Real Heroes us voluntary workers."

54. 444

The American physician and Air Force Colonel
Marcus Cranston runs in Helsinki 4 miles in the
evening, 23.4.2014 as part of a global Run-the-
World 4 Parkinson's campaign.

After receiving the diagnosis of Parkinson's disease
Cranston wanted to face the tough physical challenge and
at the same time raise money for research into
Parkinson's disease. Cranston's project combines tourism
and sport in the efforts to collect money for Michael J.
Fox Foundation. Cranston hopes to increase awareness of
the disease and to tell the stories affected by the disease.

Since 04/04/2014 Cranston has been running four miles
in 44 countries in four weeks and four days. His journey
will take to run in Asia, Australia, the Middle East, Europe
and Africa before he returns home in Las Vegas. Number
four has a significant role in the project, as Cranston's
Parkinson's disease was diagnosed when he was 44 years
old. April, the fourth month, is also the theme month of
Parkinson's disease.

Cranston seeks to demonstrate that in spite of the
diagnosis of Parkinson's disease you can continue to face
challenges of health by engaging in physical activity, by
traveling, and even acting in the armed forces.

Along the way, Marcus Cranston considered a number of
performances during which he hopes to get audiences to
connect and to share experiences. In addition, he hopes

to learn from people he meets in order to understand better the unique challenges that encounter with Parkinson's disease in different countries around the world.

Through his operation Cranston hopes also express economic support for those who wish to participate in the 4th World Parkinson Congress, which will be held in Portland, Oregon (USA) in September 2016.

Oiva club organizes activities for Marcus Cranston during his run and invites partners to co-operation. The four mile run's time of departure is at 20.00 and the place is the office of Parkinson's Association of Southern Finland. We have time to talk with Marcus Cranston before the run and after too.

Marcus Cranston wrote in the report of the visit in Finland with a title "Finland – Heroes." **Paavo Nurmi** and **Jean Sibelius** were mentioned as national heroes, but Cranston lifted up as the Real Heroes us voluntary workers.

Mark is now running the 44th 4 miles in Las Vegas. He made earlier in the journey a route change, skipped one country and added after London to the end Las Vegas, the home city.

55. All Kinds of Things Happen

I **escaped a wolf, a bear came** in front of me. This is a version of Finnish saying. And here is a solution of it. Just when I decided, after couple of weeks head scratching. that I do not after all seek full disability pension, employer University of Helsinki surprised by inviting all the 169 employees of Training and Development Center Palmenia to determination negotiations. Reduction is not more than 80 persons, so if this is the case, about half of us must leave.

U **niversity of Helsinki** kicks out the brand builder, who has during last fifteen years heard many times that he is devoted to his job, he is a key person, he is the one who is operating with new methods and technics bravely and creatively among the best developers of e-learning.

I was made redundant with six months' notice. It was as I had suspected for a long time and waited. As a result of the negotiations University of Helsinki terminates my labor relationship. Functions will be reorganized. The Palmenia Writing Program will be abolished. My work has thus reduced "substantially and permanently." The University does not offer other work or training.

Applying for a job at my age (57) and in this condition (Parkinson's diagnosis 9 years ago) does not attempt at all. I have been able to do the current job, because I have experienced it as my life's mission. Furthermore, Palmenia Writing Program is largely my own creation, which I have faithfully developed for years.

The last couple of years have been hard-pressed. I have been on a partial disability pension for over six years and received levodopa therapy more than five years. I've been in pretty good health, and I've been able to do many things I couldn't imagine when I was diagnosed, published books and travelled and done voluntary work.

Well, after half a year's notice I will have more time to these entertainments. I'm going to apply for a full disability pension after the turn of the year, and I hope that I could go straight from a partial to full disability pension without sick leave or unemployment.

P lenty to do. As an advocate of 4. World Parkinson Congress my task is to keep up the point of view of those with Parkinson's disease and their caregivers, and of course to market the WPC2016.

In addition to this, of course, there is going on book projects, one novel and one nonfiction.

T he obligation to work ended about a month ago, November 17, 2014. Ever since I have prepared to move my home, and then done it at the first week of December. There are still lamps to assemble, tables and shelves and all that stuff to put in right places.

I moved back together with my family to Malmi suburb area near the flat where my wife and daughter lived. And now we are back together. Life is unpredictable. I talked about this with a taxi driver. He said that there is no such thing like a manual in life, anything can happen He had already finished "entrepreneurial", he had changed the IT expert tasks to taxi driver and let the days to come as they came.

We have four rooms and sauna, bathroom and two toilets, a balcony, huge view because the apartment is on the 6th floor which is the top floor. So, you probably remember that we broke up last year. I needed distance. And I needed independent life.

"Parkinson icon? Me?"

- Confessions
- Searching For a New Identity

"Language is an enemy, whom you talk on your side. So is Parkinson's."

56. Confessions

Here are my confessions, written August 1, 2015, for the need of World Parkinson Coalition. The method was to complete given sentences from 45 different items.

1. PD makes me feel clumsy.

2. Because of PD, I am more aware the limits of life.

3. The reality is too painful to keep in mind all the time, especially the future, ten or fifteen years from this moment, ten year after diagnosis.

4. Before PD I suffered lack of meaning of life.

5. Now with PD I have a purpose.

6. Life is unpredictable.

7. There will never be a day that I don't think that I'm a person with Parkinson's.

8. It's hard to convince others that I don't suffer all the time.

9. It's easy to forget PD when I'm concentrated to do things I love.

10. My body is somewhat strange to me.

11. My mind is clear.

12. My heart is warmer than before PD.

13. Because of PD, my family has split once but now we are together again.

14. When I started to attend some supportive groups, I began to do voluntary work very soon.

15. My worst fear is to lose totally the control of my body.

16. Every day I look forward to scientist find out the cure.

17. I'm inspired by Michael J. Fox and other PD ambassadors with a vision.

18. If it wasn't for some co-operative volunteers in Parkinson's scene in Finland, I wouldn't have the strength to search and get two years funding for a project of people with Parkinson's at working age.

19. Now I know life is a very short flash of feeling of existence.

20. I look forward to the day I can say this all was worth it.

21. If I had one wish, it would be finding a cure for Parkinson's.

22. The biggest challenge of living with PD is to keep my mind positive, active and friendly.

23. I want to be able to handle the daily routines independently as long as possible.

24. At this moment I am feeling quite happy, because there are many new affairs in my life.

25. If I could come face to face with PD, I would say: "Bugger off!"

26. My relationship with PD is more cognitive than emotional.

27. Yesterday I felt very tired, when I was trying to go out shopping. I took my medicine and rested an hour before I left home in a better condition.

28. Today I feel energy streaming in my brain and body!

29. Tomorrow I hope I can spent a good time together with my family.

30. The main thing that has helped me feel better is medication, absolutely.

31. If there's anything I need now more than ever it is love and tenderness.

32. I'm scared because my wife will not take care of me if I'm not capable to take care of myself.

33. I'm confident because my symptoms do not develop as fast as I thought when I got diagnosis.

34. I feel like my body is someone else.

35. I feel like my mind is the true me.

36. My occupation is now a writer. Because of PD I write books faster than before.

37. My lifestyle is now very home oriented. Because of PD I spent less time outdoors than before.

38. I was diagnosed in 2005, at the age of 48, but I had clear symptoms year or two before that.

39. If only I could live a good life also alter the age of 60 – I'm 58 now.

40. The PD community is variable, contradictory and arguing – so it is as any other community.

41. The PD community needs global communication to gather the best practices to help people living with Parkinson's and especially to put together all the facilities to find the cure.

42. The people I know with PD are usually very friendly and warm hearted.

43. My doctor treats me with respect. He says "AWESOME", when I tell him about my voluntary work and medical experiments.

44. When people see my symptoms, they usually don't say anything, but kids look at me like I was a mad man!

45. The symptom that I find the worst to deal with is tremor. Right now I'm suffering it. Time to take levodopa.

57. Searching For a New Identity

Who am I? What am I? No matter how much I should be autobiographical and honest, not everything can come up talking about and there is always something one does not want to tell. The author defines always something off. I'll tell you finally some issues that are relevant to me, but which I have so far failed to tell.

This year 2015 is going to be one of the most crucial in my life. Nearly 15 years I have been working at the University of Helsinki. This has given me a solid identity of a planning officer and teacher of creative writing.

Now this identity has been taken away from me. I'm kind of naked man. What's left? Well, I am still father, husband, writer, Parkinson's activist...

Is this not enough? It should be, but does it feel like it?

I'm thinking of applying for approval today. I scanned some interviews from magazines to my computer and it came to mind, that why I agree to an open-minded interviews. Would it not be enough that I write open minded books?

I thought that if it is the approval what I search. As if I wanted to cry out: "Look at me! Embrace me with my errors even if I try for perfection."

Parkinson icon? **Me?** Adequate question. In the background of my book, unspoken, is the question: Do I want to be a Parkinson Icon as the Finnish rapper **Signmark** is the sign language icon, the wheelchair roller **Leo-Pekka Tähti** is the handicapped icon and the artist **Tom of Finland** is a homo icon. I have wanted to become an icon, or something like that, enterprise, sometimes hard working, but also the reluctance and the withdrawal from the joint action and publicity.

Iconic solidification is not as important as is the fact that interviews and other public activities do bring out the positive images from Parkinson's disease. The whole picture of the disease is not at all the late stage suffering. Journalists and the media in general make a real contribution here. Stories and headlines occupy positive message for general public:

- Hand is clumsy - imagination is not
- Familiar Parkinson's
- My life became rich
- Parkinson's taught to live

Two deaths lately. My oldest cousin and the cousin of my mother. Each morning that I wake up to a new day is a miracle!

Everything is possible! Magnitude and seeing meanings. Must struggle that realities remain. If there exist any reality in the near future of me! After all everything is possible! I wonder if I have hypomania, a mild mania, now that the job is going to expire next week. I get a lot of new ideas and make interpretations of premarks.

This is totally out of topic, but I have to tell you, that I wrote the other day in Facebook to John Irving as follows: "Thank you for honoring the great German author fellow, who passed away recently. Here in Finland we read Günter Grass with pleasure and intellectual curiosity as we read you, John Irving. It is interesting what you tell about Grass as one of your teachers – I must say that you have been a source of creativity and inspiration for many of us who have a passion to write novels and short stories, not to mention reading them."

Now I read that note differently. It's question of memorizing your dear ones.

Yesterday was the international Parkinson's day. To celebrate it I had intended to write a blog post. But what happened? I was all day so exhausted that I just scribbled in a notebook sketches of advanced Parkinson's seminar in Finlandia Hall the day before.

I have used in this book words, which I have not known before – proposed by machine translators and accepted by me in good faith. I have taken risks. To a native speaker my words can be strange. To me they are only visitors, whom I let come in in spite of the threat of violence. You know, language is an enemy, whom you talk on your side. So is Parkinson's.

Contact

Comment? Questions?

Please, contact me if there is something you want to share.

montonentimo13@gmail.com

http://timomontonen.jimdo.com/

http://www.parkinsontyossa.fi/

https://www.facebook.com/timo.montonen

Notes